JOHN STEAKLEY

Rhythms of Recovery

Finding the Rhythm Your Heart Was Made To Follow

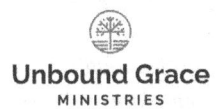

First published by Unbound Grace Ministries 2025

Copyright © 2025 by John Steakley

All rights reserved. No part of this publication may be reproduced, stored or transmitted in any form or by any means, electronic, mechanical, photocopying, recording, scanning, or otherwise without written permission from the publisher. It is illegal to copy this book, post it to a website, or distribute it by any other means without permission.

John Steakley asserts the moral right to be identified as the author of this work.

John Steakley has no responsibility for the persistence or accuracy of URLs for external or third-party Internet Websites referred to in this publication and does not guarantee that any content on such Websites is, or will remain, accurate or appropriate.

Designations used by companies to distinguish their products are often claimed as trademarks. All brand names and product names used in this book and on its cover are trade names, service marks, trademarks and registered trademarks of their respective owners. The publishers and the book are not associated with any product or vendor mentioned in this book. None of the companies referenced within the book have endorsed the book.

First edition

ISBN: 979-8-9932035-0-8

Editing by George Edema, Tyler Harris, Cameron Patterson, Lauren Middlebrooks, Karen Bouchard
Cover art by Lauren Middlebrooks

*This book was professionally typeset on Reedsy.
Find out more at reedsy.com*

Contents

Introduction   vi
Your Commitment   x

I   Honesty

1	Day 1 - Honesty With Self	3
2	Day 2 - Justice and Honesty	6
3	Day 3 - Honesty, Sovereignty & Acceptance	10
4	Day 4 - Honesty: Living Free Instead of Dying Hard	15

II   Humility

5	Day 1 - The Humble Soul	23
6	Day 2 - "I'm So Humble"	28
7	Day 3 - Put on Humility	34
8	Day 4 - Christ's Humility	39

III   Repentance

9	Day 1 - Repentance is an Invitation	45
10	Day 2 - Rhythms of Repentance	50
11	Day 3 - Repentance & Rest for Your Soul	55
12	Day 4 - A Repentance Letter	60

IV Gratitude

13	Day 1 – What is Gratitude?	67
14	Day 2 – Thanksgiving vs. Anxiety	71
15	Day 3 – Locked Up & Thankful	75
16	Day 4 – Entitlement: A "Screwtape" Letter	78

V Forgiveness

17	Day 1 – The Waterfall of Forgiveness	85
18	Day 2 – Extending Forgiveness	89
19	Day 3 – The Cost and Power of Forgiveness	93
20	Day 4 – Revenge: A "Screwtape" Letter	97

VI Spiritual Disciplines

21	Day 1 – Spiritual Discipline	105
22	Day 2 – God's Word to Humanity	110
23	Day 3 – The Privilege of Prayer	115
24	Day 4 – Freedom to Worship	119

VII Peace & Patience

25	Day 1 – Shalom in the Hurricane	127
26	Day 2 – Practicing Peace	131
27	Day 3 – Active Patience	136
28	Day 4 – Patience: A "Screwtape" Letter	140

VIII Obedience & Self-Control

29	Day 1 - Obedience: Submission to God's Authority	147
30	Day 2 - Obedience from Love	151
31	Day 3 - Self-Control: Sustained Obedience	155
32	Day 4 - Obedience & Self-Control: A "Screwtape" Letter	159

IX Love

33	Day 1 - God is Love, Part 1	167
34	Day 2 - God is Love, Part 2: A Transformative Example	171
35	Day 3 - Love Your Enemies? Seriously?	175
36	Day 4 - Love in Action	178

X Worship & Christian Community

37	Day 1 - Worship: The Rhythm of Recovery	183
38	Day 2 - The Lord's Day	188
39	Day 3 - All of Life as Worship	193
40	Day 4 - Together	198

About the Author	202
Also by John Steakley	204

Introduction

Preserve me, O God, for in you I take refuge. I say to the Lord, "You are my Lord; I have no good apart from you."... You make known to me the path of life; in your presence there is fullness of joy; at your right hand are pleasures forevermore.
Psalm 16 (*ESV*)

What is this book?

This book is for anyone seeking hope, healing, or deeper connection. It's designed to be used by individuals or groups—whether you're in a season of recovery, growth, or simply looking to engage more deeply with your faith and story. We encourage you to go through it with a friend, mentor, small group, or someone you trust in your community. You don't have to walk this journey alone.

Together in Recovery

Addiction affects everyone. Addiction is not an unfamiliar concept relegated to the fringes of society; it is the uninvited house guest within the hallways of our hearts, a testament to our fallen nature.

Our endeavor here is not just sobriety (a state of mere abstention) but a comprehensive, all-encompassing spiritual health. It is about learning to depend on God, abide in Him, and tap into the deep reservoir of His grace that leads to genuine, lasting transformation. The emphasis of this journey is not merely behavioral change but a transformation that affects every facet of life.

And so, this book isn't exclusively for those wrestling with what the world labels as "addictions." It is for every single one of us. If we are honest, haven't we all tasted the bitterness of doing what we don't want to do, and not doing what we yearn to do? The Apostle Paul himself resonated with this struggle, penning the paradox of our shared human experience.

This book is a compass, a road map, and a companion in our shared journey of recovery. If you are a follower of Jesus, you may have discovered that you are in the midst of this recovery journey: *recovering from a past life of emptiness and enslavement to sin, and learning to navigate the narrow path to abundant life in faith and dependency on Christ Jesus.*

This workbook takes you on a ten-week journey, each week taking a step further into the themes central to our recovery:

Week 1: Honesty
Week 2: Humility
Week 3: Repentance
Week 4: Gratitude
Week 5: Forgiveness
Week 6: Spiritual Disciplines
Week 7: Peace & Patience
Week 8: Self-control & Obedience

Week 9: Love
Week 10: Worship & Christian Community

Weekly Rhythms

1. READ. Every week, you'll be asked to read four brief readings and take a simple action step to begin creating new rhythms in your life. The week will culminate in a meeting with your mentor/group—please read the material before each meeting.

2. ANSWER. Each reading includes interactive questions. Write your answers down and be ready to share your thoughts with your group.

3. SHARE. During each weekly meeting, you and your group will walk through that week's material together, using your answers to the interactive questions for discussion and encouragement.

4. IMPLEMENT. Throughout your recovery journey, continue implementing what you learn. As you practice what you've learned, new habits will begin to form, and the concepts discussed will become part of who you are.

We believe that mere sobriety falls short of the abundant life our Creator desires for us. These readings are *not* about performance or checking off tasks; they are about embracing the freedom to move beyond the enslavement of addiction and into the abundant life our Creator desires for us.

Additional Tools & Resources

If you are looking for more support on your recovery journey, check out John Steakley's book, *Unbound Grace: Hope in the Wilderness of Addiction,* which includes several practical tools that complement this workbook. You can find more information on our website, https://unboundgrace.life.

Getting Started

This is real life. It is walking together, learning to rely on God, His word, and genuine fellowship. It's about setting up a path to recovery that is purposeful, accessible, transformational, and faithful.

This journey will demand courage, humility, and a willingness to step into uncharted lands, but *you do not walk alone.* You have access to someone who is walking with you—not just your mentor/group, but God Himself—and together you can face your enemies and taste the victory of faith.

Respond to the call. Step onto this path of freedom, where we can travel, grow, and heal together. And may this book serve as a lighthouse in your journey toward spiritual and emotional recovery.

Your Commitment

Do I Dare Commit?

Don't think of this workbook (or other recovery tools) as the key to a perfect and flawless recovery. In fact, it's possible to use new life rhythms or recovery tools to fake it for a while—but eventually the truth will out you. Instead, think of these weekly rhythms as signposts leading you out of the wilderness of addiction toward spiritual health, as your guide to a faithful and life-giving recovery.

This workbook is designed to promote healthy community, encourage your clear and sacred identity, and provide signposts for spiritual growth. It is designed to foster positive behaviors that will move you *away from* addiction by leading you *toward* true life. In these pages, you will not find lists of rules and prohibitions but a path out of the wilderness of addiction into healthy recovery in community.

Are you willing to commit to these rhythms of life each week?
Will you dare to move away from the sin that entangles you and begin to trust that God will provide you freedom from your struggle? Will you trust God with the hidden parts of your life? Will you trust others to come alongside you in this battle?

Remember, this journey is about grace over works and faithfulness over performance. It's not about checking off tasks but embracing a transformation that leads to true freedom and peace. Are you ready to take the first step? Let's begin.

Your Commitment:

I, _____ (your name), commit to reading this book, not rushing through all at once, but processing the readings thoughtfully throughout each week—to the best of my ability.

I commit to share my journey with (at least one friend):

Name:_____

Name:_____

Name:_____

We commit to meeting weekly at _____ (time) at _____ (place) to the best of our abilities.

I commit to honesty and faithfulness as I embark on this journey of recovery.

Sign:_____

Date:_____

I

Honesty

Day 1 - **Honesty with Self**

Day 2 - **Justice and Honesty**

Day 3 - **Honesty, Sovereignty & Acceptance**

Day 4 - **Honesty: Living Free Instead of Dying Hard**

1

Day 1 - Honesty With Self

What good would it do to get everything you want and lose you, the real you? What could you ever trade your soul for?
Mark 8:36-37 (MSG)

In the shadows of addiction, we are enslaved to self-deception and lying to others. Recovery begins in the light of honesty. In recovery, we are free to be honest with ourselves and others.

When I was in rehab, one of the men in my processing group said he always knew he was close to relapsing when he would become dishonest about small, seemingly trivial things.

"I would lie about the dumbest things. I would go to Burger King and tell my wife I went to McDonald's. Or I would run into a friend at the store and tell him I had just returned from vacation when I had not been on vacation. When the lies started coming automatically, it was only a matter of time before I relapsed."

His lies to himself and others were more than a precursor to relapse. They were intrinsic to his entrapment. This was his eleventh stint in rehab. In the first ten rehabs, he was never honest with himself or others. But during his eleventh rehab, he realized that alcohol was literally killing him, and he decided to take it seriously. For the first time in his life, he had the courage to be honest with himself.

When we are dishonest, we present a fake version of ourselves to the world. Over time, we can even begin to believe our own lies. This is the nature of addiction. The insane thing about dishonesty is that both you and God know you are lying, and there is a good chance that the people you are trying to deceive know too.

If you follow Jesus, you have been released from the need to lie. Because of Jesus, you have a new identity. You are his child, and nothing can change that. When He looks at you, he no longer sees your sin, He sees Christ's righteousness covering you.

> *"If I speak what is false, I must answer for it;*
> *if true, it will answer for me."*
> *-Thomas Fuller*

* * *

Write Your Thoughts

- How does it make you feel when someone lies to you? How have your lies hurt others in the past?

- In what situations are you tempted to lie? Why?

- What does it look like to be completely honest with yourself? Is this difficult or easy for you?

Create A New Rhythm

This week, if/when you feel tempted to lie or embellish the truth, try to stop and ask yourself, "What do I really want?" Compare the "lies" that you want to say or think with the truth. Once you identify the truth, pray that God will help you to be honest with yourself and honest with others.

> *So Jesus said to the Jews who had believed him, "If you abide in my word, you are truly my disciples, and you will know the truth, and the truth will set you free."*
> John 8:31-32 (ESV)

2

Day 2 - Justice and Honesty

*A false balance is an abomination to the LORD,
but a just weight is his delight.*
Proverbs 11:1 (ESV)

Elizabeth Holmes, the world's youngest female self-made billionaire, founded Theranos in 2003. Her company promised to revolutionize the medical industry by developing a device that could run various diagnostic tests from a few drops of blood.

Holmes proudly claimed that the U.S. Department of Defense was utilizing Theranos' technology on the battlefield and that her company was revolutionizing the medical industry. Theranos raised hundreds of millions of dollars, reaching a valuation of $9 billion at its peak.

Holmes is currently serving an 11-year prison sentence for the lies she told about her company. As it turns out, Theranos never even built the blood testing machine that she claimed was so revolutionary. In addition to serving time in prison, Holmes was also ordered to pay almost half a billion dollars in restitution.

Have you ever lied to look good or get ahead in life? We all have our own scales. We might not be leading billion-dollar companies, but we are all capable of tipping the balance dishonestly in our favor in the little day-to-day transactions of life. It might be as simple as a white lie, an embellished story, or even dodging personal responsibility. In every dishonest act, we shift the weight of truth to create a false balance, a disgrace in the eyes of the Lord.

In addiction, we often encounter false scales. Maybe we deny the extent of our struggle or our need for help. This creates a false balance. But like Theranos, the truth has a way of surfacing and exposing the lies. *Recovery begins with honesty and admitting our struggles.* This process aligns with the 'just weight' that delights the Lord.

Just as God delights in an honest weight, He also delights in an honest heart. Our challenge is to live with integrity and embrace a life of rigorous honesty. As we do so, we can trust that God, in His grace, will help us maintain a balance that is true, just, and pleasing to Him.

* * *

Write Your Thoughts

- How does the story of Elizabeth Holmes illuminate the principle in Proverbs 11:1 (found at the beginning of this chapter), and how can this principle be applied to our daily lives?

- How does dishonesty manifest in different areas of life, such as in our personal relationships or during the process of recovery?

- What does it mean to maintain an "honest weight" in the context of our beliefs, responsibilities, and struggles? Can you think of any examples from your own life?

- How does recognizing God's sovereignty encourage honesty and integrity, and what practical steps can we take to align ourselves with this principle?

Create a New Rhythm

DAY 2 - JUSTICE AND HONESTY

Take a few minutes to pray and ask God to reveal any areas in your life where you have been dishonest, or are being dishonest with yourself, with others, or even with God. He loves you and already knows the truth. Ask God to help you accept the truth, and to be honest with yourself and others.

3

Day 3 - Honesty, Sovereignty & Acceptance

Whatever the Lord pleases, he does, in heaven and on earth, in the seas and all deeps. He it is who makes the clouds rise at the end of the earth, who makes lightning for the rain and brings forth the wind from his storehouses.
Psalm 135:6-7 (ESV)

The definition of sovereignty is "supreme power or authority." In Christianity, God is sovereign, meaning He reigns over all and His will is the ultimate rule of all things. Nothing happens outside of God's control. He is the Creator and the Sustainer. As his beloved image-bearing creatures, we get to enjoy the freedom that comes from knowing and walking with our good and sovereign king. "The Lord is my shepherd."

Consider the faithful believers of the Old Testament and the New Testament's early church. Instead of being anxious about earning favor on their own strength, or grasping for control over their lives and the lives of others, these men and women trusted and rested in God's sovereignty over everything. Their lives shined brightly: bold, free, and beautiful, even through extreme trials.

To shine with this same light, to live with this same bold freedom, we must truly rest in the same sovereign hands of God. To grow in recovery, we embrace and accept that God is in control, not us. When we embrace this, we are freed from the insanity of trying to be in control. This acceptance of God's sovereignty and our own limitations extends to how we view our story, our struggles, and the people God has placed in our lives.

The fourth edition of the "Big Book" of Alcoholics Anonymous has a famous section on acceptance. In the passage, the author writes that he has come to realize that in order to live with any sort of contentment, he must accept the realities of life. The author writes,

> And acceptance is the answer to all my problems today. When I am disturbed, it is because I find some person, place, thing, or situation – some fact of my life – unacceptable to me, and I can find no serenity until I accept that person, place, thing, or situation as being exactly the way it is supposed to be at this moment.

In this life, we feel pressure all around us. Many of these things are legitimate problems and cause legitimate suffering. Acceptance doesn't mean we are fatalists and refuse to seek the good and protect against the bad. It means that our faith is grounded in the understanding that God has command over all situations and is actively present in our lives. The challenges we are presently navigating are the exact circumstances intended for us to affirm and deepen our trust in Him at this moment.

The Big Book author notes, "When I complain about me or about you, I am complaining about God's handiwork. I am saying that I know better than God." Acceptance is often not easy. And we need the help of our sovereign King. Just as we are all equally in need of rescue by our Savior, we also must be rescued from our desire to control our lives and deny God's sovereignty. Our acceptance of the truth that God is in control and we are not is intimately bound to our dependence upon him and not on ourselves.

When I consider my own journey honestly, I would not go back and change my struggle with alcohol and pills. That struggle was one of the best gifts God has given me. It has revealed how deeply I need him and how lost I am on my own. I would never choose addiction, but it has directed me to depend on Christ and rest in the sovereign care of God.

I think these two equations sum it up beautifully:

The Desire for Control + Nonacceptance =
Rejection of Peace (Serenity)

God's Control + Acceptance =
Freedom and Peace

If God is truly Lord over creation, then he is in complete control over all things. His sovereign power is not impersonal or uncaring but is instead the loving and gracious rule of the king

DAY 3 - HONESTY, SOVEREIGNTY & ACCEPTANCE

of creation and redemption. The key to acceptance, then, is acknowledging that he is in control and is more loving, wise, and powerful than we can imagine.

* * *

Write Your Thoughts

- Look again at Psalm 135. What kinds of things do you observe in your life that inspire you to reflect on the sovereign grace of God?

- Do you recall a time when you rested in the hands of the sovereign God? If so, what do you remember about it? If not, have you seen that rest in others? What did it look like?

- What are you struggling to accept today? (Be specific, be detailed)

- Do you have an example of how acceptance has brought you freedom? If not, what do you think this looks like in real life?

Create a New Rhythm

Grasping for control is a disease passed down by the Fall. Acceptance isn't giving up; it's resting in the grace of the One who gave Himself for us. In trusting God, we find peace that the world can't take away.

4

Day 4 - Honesty: Living Free Instead of Dying Hard

> *We know that we are held firm by God; it's only the people who do not follow Jesus that continue in the grip of the Evil One. And we know that the Son of God came so we could recognize and understand the truth of God—what a gift!—and we are living in the Truth itself, in God's Son, Jesus Christ. This Jesus is both True God and Real Life.*
> 1 John 5:18-20 (MSG)

Why do we lie? Lying is a defense mechanism that (superficially) prevents us from revealing our true selves to another person. This allows us to create a false sense of control and safety. Maybe we are trying to save face, avoid hurting someone, impress, avoid responsibility, hide shame, or prevent tension with others.

It can be so easy to justify or excuse our lies. But drastic honesty is essential to spiritual and relational health. Telling the truth, even when it makes us look bad, helps us to be conscious of and accountable for our actions. It also creates a fertile environment for intimacy with others as we build trust.

Telling the truth brings freedom. Jesus said that "If you abide in my word, you are truly my disciples, and you will know the truth, and the truth will set you free" (John 8:31-32). Telling the truth about our lives and our problems to another person allows us to see them clearly. When we start speaking the truth about our lives and our problems, not only to others but also to ourselves, it's as if we've emerged from the cave into the sunlight. God's truth, once we embrace it, has the power to set us free from the cold and shadowy cave of deception. As we venture outside into the light, we see the world for what it is, rather than being lost in the distorted shadows of dishonesty.

We often lie reflexively, especially in addiction. Our dishonesty becomes so ingrained in us that we lie without thinking about it. We're so inwardly focused on selfish, immediate desires that we don't stop to consider the consequences.

When we tell a lie or allow someone to believe something about us that is untrue, we create a cloak of lies that we must now wear everywhere we go. Over time, we are forced to reinforce the cloak with layer after layer as we cover our tracks with more lies. The instant gratification of a lie seems satisfying, but over time, it is either discovered or becomes a monster that dominates our lives.

It's time to lay down our burden of dishonesty and burn that cloak. Life in recovery must have a foundation of honesty. True sobriety, both emotional and physical, requires truth-telling.

Being honest feels risky. Many of us are afraid to be honest, feeling that if people knew our character flaws, they would not like us or think less of us. Ironically, most of the time, the opposite is true. The vulnerability we show by exposing our imperfections allows people to come closer to us. This is because our shortcomings tend to mirror their own, and by revealing our true selves, we help them connect and belong.

This kind of sharing creates a sense of safety. When others are honest with us about their shortcomings, we feel safe to be ourselves around them. We are secure enough in that relationship to be who we are, without feeling the need to hide. This kind of openness is crucial to have meaningful relationships in our lives. More than that, our honesty points to our creator.

> *"Son, you can be impressive or you can be known, but you can't be both."*
> *- Ray Ortlund*

* * *

Write Your Thoughts

- Give an example of a lie you told in active addiction. What was the outcome of telling this lie?

- How does being honest affect our relationships, especially when it makes us look bad?

- What does Jesus mean when he says, "I am the way, and the truth, and the life. No one comes to the Father except through me" (John 14:6 *ESV*)?

- When Jesus says, "the truth will set you free," what truth is he referring to?

Create a New Rhythm

We don't have to duck into the shadows—
   Jesus already sees us, and still He stays.
   We tell the truth, not to impress, but because
   He *is* the Truth, and He holds us steady.
   We drop the lies, every excuse, every cover-up, because
   He carried the whole weight of our shame on His shoulders.
   Now we walk in the light, not to look good, but to live free.

DAY 4 - HONESTY: LIVING FREE INSTEAD OF DYING HARD

Telling the truth isn't easy.
   But it's honest.
   It's holy.
   And with Jesus, it's safe.

II

Humility

Day 1 - ***The Humble Soul***

Day 2 - ***"I'm So Humble"***

Day 3 - ***Put On Humility***

Day 4 - ***Christ's Humility***

5

Day 1 - The Humble Soul

If you puff yourself up, you'll get the wind knocked out of you. But if you're content to simply be yourself, your life will count for plenty.
Matthew 23:12 (MSG)

My closest friend was recently promoted to CEO of his company. It was a big deal. He loves his company and believes in the people he works with. When he called to tell me the news, he was excited yet humble. When we met up a week later, he told me how his daughters reacted to hearing about his promotion.

His daughters were playing in the yard on a beautiful spring day after a string of bad weather. My friend joined them, and as they kicked the soccer ball together, he told them about the promotion. That's when, in a forthright and matter-of-fact way, one of his twins said, "Dad, who cares? Let's just play."

He told me he just kind of laughed to himself and did exactly what she requested; he kept playing with his girls. Later that night, as they were doing their bedtime routine, the same daughter who brushed off his big news told him how proud she was of him, and that he was already very special to her, no matter what his job was.

At his daughter's initial reaction to his announcement, my friend could have been upset and tried to explain what a big deal the promotion was. Instead, he decided to enjoy their time together and not think twice about it.

This father/daughter interaction leads to some important questions: What is humility? What does it mean to be humble? What is the mindset of the humble soul?

Philippians 2:3 (*ESV*)

> Do nothing from selfish ambition or conceit, but in humility count others as more significant than yourselves.

Tim Keller said, "The essence of gospel humility is not thinking more of myself or thinking less of myself, *it is thinking of myself less.*" In other words, humility is sort of like forgetting to focus on yourself. It's the "Who cares? Let's just play," sort of mindset.

Humility is having the correct view of ourselves in relation to God and others, and then acting accordingly. A person cannot have a correct view of themselves without God. God is love, and his love leads to humility because it helps us see how completely dependent we are on him and his grace.

Your heart beats over 100,000 times a day. Each pump of

DAY 1 - THE HUMBLE SOUL

your heart is the beat of God's grace. Consider your next breath. What did you do to earn this gift? Nothing. Your life and every good thing you experience are a gift from God, and every bad experience is an opportunity to run to him for security, comfort, and purpose.

A straightforward definition of grace is "God's undeserved, unearned favor, given freely to the unworthy." And it is counter to the mindset of the world. The world's wisdom tells people to earn their place in society – to work harder, and then they will reap the rewards of their effort and success. From the world's viewpoint, true humility is foolish, costly, and weak. In God's economy, however, humility brings peace and contentment.

The seventh step of Alcoholics Anonymous (AA) has some great wisdom on humility. It is about changing your attitude and moving forward with humility so you can give yourself over to God and ask him to do what you cannot do on your own: rid yourself of the faults that have harmed yourself and others.

Take a moment to reflect on the Seventh Step Prayer:

> *My Creator, I am now willing that you should have all of me, good and bad. I pray that you now remove from me every single defect of character which stands in the way of my usefulness to you and my fellows. Grant me strength, as I go out from here, to do your bidding. Amen. (Alcoholics Anonymous book, page 76).*

* * *

Write Your Thoughts

- John Flavel wrote, "They that know God, will be humble; they that know themselves, cannot be proud." In your opinion, what is the link between knowing ourselves and humility?

- According to Tim Keller, what is humility?

- How did the father in the illustration model humility?

- Do you give God credit for how far you have come? If not, why not? If yes, how should that change the way you live your life?

Create a New Rhythm

The next time you have an opportunity to brag, respond with humility by expressing thankfulness to God instead.

6

Day 2 - "I'm So Humble"

Before I was afflicted I went astray, but now I keep your word... It is good for me that I was afflicted, that I might learn your statutes... I know, O Lord, that your rules are righteous, and that in faithfulness you have afflicted me... If your law had not been my delight, I would have perished in my affliction... Your word is a lamp to my feet and a light to my path.
Psalm 119:67, 71, 75, 92, 105 (ESV)

Dick Bass was an adventurer. One of his greatest feats is being the first person to climb the highest peak on each of the seven continents. He was also the oldest person, at the age of 55, to climb Mount Everest.

He had a reputation for sharing his adventures with anyone who would listen. On one particular occasion, he sat down on a plane and began to share his death-defying stories with the nice man sitting next to him. He shared about summiting the beautiful and deadly peaks of Mt. McKinley and Mt. Everest and his near-death experience in the Himalayas.

As the plane was about to land, he realized he had never introduced himself to the man he had been talking to the entire flight, so he leaned over and said, "My name is Dick Bass. Pleased to meet you."

The kind man shook his hand and answered, "Hello, my name is Neil Armstrong. It is nice to meet you." [1]

Can you imagine the moment when Dick Bass realized he could have spent the entire flight talking to the first person to walk on the moon about space travel and Armstrong's unrepeatable feat? Instead, he spent the entire time talking about himself. Armstrong, however, displayed humility by not focusing on himself. I wonder if Dick Bass ever compared his pride with Neil Armstrong's humility.

Most of us have moments when we act like Mr. Bass. We have promoted ourselves instead of walking the path of humility. Only God knows what we have missed as a result of our pride.

We like to surround ourselves with a house of mirrors. Consider, for example, social media - a platform to constantly promote ourselves and satisfy our ego. We are surrounded by self-promotion so much that true humility stands out when we encounter it.

So, what does it look like to walk in humility versus walking in pride? What does the Bible promise about walking in humility?

---

[1] Roger Horchow and Sally Horchow, *The Art of Friendship: 70 Simple Rules for Making Meaningful Connections* (New York: St. Martin's Press, 2006).

Humility vs. Pride

Humility is the mindset of complete dependence on God for anything good and the complete insufficiency of one's efforts. Humility is a recognition of God's grace.

Humility:

- Asks for help
- Is the posture of prayer (looking to the Creator for direction in life)
- Is self-aware
- Is compassionate
- Does not judge
- Requires no self-defense
- Listens when interrupted
- Listens actively
- Is open to learning from others

Pride:

- Doesn't ask for help
- Prays a list of wants
- Exalts self
- Does not fear the Lord.
- Blocks out emotions
- Always judges
- Knows everything about humility except how to practice it
- Insists on its way
- Refuses to learn from others

DAY 2 - "I'M SO HUMBLE"

The Promises of Humility & Consequences of Pride

Humility promises:

- Humility comes before honor (Proverbs 18:12, 15:33)
- Wisdom (Proverbs 11:2)
- Forgiveness and healing (2 Chronicles 7:14)
- God's grace (James 4:6; Proverbs 3:34; Isaiah 66:2)
- Knowledge of God's way (Psalm 25:9)
- Rest for your souls (Matthew 11:29-30)

Consequences of Pride:

- Disgrace (Proverbs 11:2)
- God's opposition (James 4:6)
- Will bring you low (Proverbs 29:23)
- Leads to destruction (Proverbs 16:18; 18:12)
- Pride deceives us (Obadiah 1:3; Galatians 6:3)

Think about the nature of pride. It is never-ending, and its false form of satisfaction is short-lived. The Bible is full of beautiful paradoxes, and humility is one of them. Humility lifts up while pride chops down. Humility brings honor and life, and pride brings ruin.

What does humility look like in action? C.S. Lewis provides a masterful description in his book *Mere Christianity*:

> Do not imagine that if you meet a really humble man he will be what most people call "humble" nowadays:

he will not be a sort of greasy, smarmy person, who is always telling you that, of course, he is nobody.

Probably all you will think about him is that he seemed a cheerful, intelligent chap who took a real interest in what you said to him. If you do dislike him it will be because you feel a little envious of anyone who seems to enjoy life so easily. He will not be thinking about humility: he will not be thinking about himself at all.[2]

* * *

Write Your Thoughts

- Review the list under the section "What is humility" and "What is pride." Which of the points from this list have you experienced before?

- Review the list under "promises of humility and consequences of pride". Which of the points from this list have you identified with before?

---

[2] C.S. Lewis, *Mere Christianity* (New York: HarperOne, 2001), 128.

- According to Tim Keller, "The Bible says the persons most quick to defend themselves are the weakest, not the strongest." What is an example of a time you have been prideful? What was the outcome of your pride?

Create a New Rhythm

According to C.S. Lewis, "For pride is spiritual cancer: it eats up the very possibility of love, or contentment, or even common sense." Pray and ask God to remove your pride and grant you humility. In fact, begin every morning by asking for humility to make it a regular part of your routine.

7

Day 3 - Put on Humility

Clothe yourselves, all of you, with humility towards one another, for "God opposes the proud but gives grace to the humble."
1 Peter 5:5 (ESV)

Everyone has encountered pride in their own heart and in others. It is a universal human problem. Everyone suffers from it. By nature, we want to look good and feel important – we want to be exalted. We want to matter to someone. We often want the praise of others so desperately that we will lie and manipulate others to get it.

C.S. Lewis warns, "Make no mistake about it: pride is the great sin. It is the Devil's most effective and destructive tool." God knows that we all experience pride—and how destructive it is to our souls and lives. He longs for our restoration and to put us in "right standing" with him. Scripture teaches that God wants restoration, not condemnation. He does not want to punish us just for the sake of punishment, but desires to forgive and restore us. But first, we must admit that we are powerless and need help.

James 4:10 (*ESV*) says, "Humble yourselves, and I will exalt you." This is the way of God's upside-down kingdom. God designed us to need him. Humility recognizes this. God delights in humility, he delights in restoration and healing, and—when we are humble before him, he delights in us! In the words of Psalm 147:11 (ESV), "The LORD delights in those who fear him, who put their hope in his unfailing love."

Paul tells us that we are to "put on then, as God's chosen ones, holy and beloved, compassionate hearts, kindness, humility, meekness, and patience" (Colossians 3:12 *ESV*). So what does it look like to "put on" or "clothe yourself" with humility? Jesus tells a story about two men in Luke 18:11-14. One is full of pride, and the other is humble. One will "end up flat on [his] face," and the other is made right with God.

> Two men went up to the Temple to pray, one a Pharisee, the other a tax man. The Pharisee posed and prayed like this: "Oh, God, I thank you that I am not like other people—robbers, crooks, adulterers, or, heaven forbid, like this tax man. I fast twice a week and tithe on all my income."
>
> Meanwhile the tax man, slumped in the shadows, his face in his hands, not daring to look up, said, "God, give mercy. Forgive me, a sinner."
>
> Jesus commented, "This tax man, not the other, went home made right with God. If you walk around with your nose in the air, you're going to end up flat on your face, but if you're content to be simply

yourself, you will become more than yourself." (Luke 18:11-14 MSG).

Notice that the religious person's prayer is not really about God but about how good he is and how wrong others are. In this story, *pride is wrapped in the cloak of religion* and gives it a bad name.

The tax collector, on the other hand, is so painfully aware of his sins and unworthiness before God that he cannot even lift his eyes as he stands in the back of the temple, far from the altar. He has put on the cloak of humility. Pounding his chest in sorrowful *contrition* over his sins, he can only manage the desperate plea, "God, be merciful to me, a sinner."

To be contrite means to feel remorseful and penitent—and it opens the way for us to experience the goodness and blessings of God. The Psalmist writes, "a broken and contrite heart, O God, you will not despise" (Psalm 51:17 ESV). And in Proverbs we read, "Pride lands you flat on your face; humility prepares you for honors" (Proverbs 29:23 MSG).

When we live humbly, we are living out our true nature. We are living the way God created us to live, aware of our need for God. We are also living out our salvation. Our salvation naturally produces humility in us because when we could not save ourselves, God, in faithful love and mercy, "took our sin-dead lives and made us alive in Christ. He did all this on his own, with no help from us! Then he picked us up and set us down in the highest heaven in company with Jesus, our Messiah" (Ephesians 2:5-6 MSG).

To "clothe [our]selves... with humility toward one another" is to remember that we can relate to both the "tax man" and the "Pharisee." We can humbly acknowledge that it is by God's grace alone that we are allowed to worship the creator of the universe.

> *For while we were still weak, at the right time Christ died for the ungodly… but God shows his love for us in that while we were still sinners, Christ died for us.*
> Romans 5:6, 8 (ESV)

* * *

Write Your Thoughts

- Why does God delight in our humility?

- Who are like most of the time, the Pharisee or the taxman?

- What does God ultimately do with those who put on "the cloak of humility"?

Create a New Rhythm

Find the area of your life where you are most like the Pharisee (proud) and ask God to give you the humility to be like the tax man.

8

Day 4 - Christ's Humility

Do nothing from selfish ambition or conceit, but in humility count others more significant than yourselves. Let each of you look not only to his own interests but also to the interests of others. Have this mind among yourselves, which is yours in Christ Jesus, who, though he was in the form of God, did not count equality with God a thing to be grasped, but emptied himself, by taking the form of a servant, being born in the likeness of men. And being found in human form, he humbled himself by becoming obedient to the point of death, even death on a cross. Therefore God has highly exalted him and bestowed on him the name that is above every name, so that at the name of Jesus every knee should bow, in heaven and on earth and under the earth, and every tongue confess that Jesus Christ is Lord, to the glory of God the Father.
Philippians 2:3-11 (ESV)

Christ, the Son of God, took on human form and walked among us, not as a powerful ruler but as a humble servant. He walked this earth as fully man and fully God. He washed his disciples' feet, ate with sinners and tax collectors, and healed the sick and the marginalized. He never sought glory for himself, but always directed attention to his heavenly Father.

In John 13, Jesus is having a final meal with his disciples before his crucifixion. During the meal, Jesus removes his outer garment, wraps a towel around his waist, and begins washing his disciples' feet. This was an act of humility, as foot washing was a task typically performed by servants. Peter initially objects to Jesus washing his feet, but Jesus explains that it is necessary to show them an example of how to serve others.

There is no more significant example of humility than Christ. By taking on human form, he willingly subjected himself to all the limitations and vulnerabilities of humanity, experiencing hunger, thirst, fatigue, and pain, as well as facing rejection, persecution, and, ultimately, a gruesome death.

Christ's humility was not weakness, but strength. It was not a negative view of himself, but a deep understanding of his mission and identity. He knew that true greatness comes from serving others, not from building himself up.

Through his humility, Christ displayed (embodied) the very essence of God's character, which is love. He humbled himself to serve and save us, and his ultimate act of self-sacrifice on the cross demonstrated the depth of his love for us. His humility is a gift to us because we are the ones who need to be washed. We are the ones who need saving. And by faith, Christ's righteous humility is given to us, as if it were our own. This is what gives us the ability to follow Christ's example and humbly serve others.

According to Andrew Murray, Christ is the "humility of God embodied in human nature".[3] Christ's example calls us to follow in his footsteps, serving one another with love and humility.

In his humility, Christ set an example for us to follow. We are called to lay down our own desires and ambitions and to serve others with love and compassion. As we do this, over time, our desires and dreams will align with Christ's. We are to imitate his sacrificial love and selflessness and to remember that our true worth comes not from what we accomplish, but from our relationship with God (what he has accomplished).

May we all receive Christ's grace, learn from the example of his humility, and strive to live as humble servants of God.

* * *

Write Your Thoughts

- Other than washing his disciples' feet, what is one example of humility from Jesus' life?

- Who did Jesus say he came to give glory to? Why?

---

[3] Andrew Murray, *Humility: The Journey Toward Holiness* (New York: Christian Literature Crusade, 1895).

- As we serve others in humility and count them more important than ourselves, what happens to our desires?

Create a New Rhythm

Find two people this week and do something to serve them, expecting nothing in return. You may be surprised by their reaction!

III

Repentance

Day 1 - **Repentance Is An Invitation**

Day 2 - **Rhythms of Repentance**

Day 3 - **Repentance & Rest for Your Soul**

Day 4 - **Psalm 51, A Repentance Letter**

9

Day 1 - Repentance is an Invitation

And I will give you a new heart, and a new spirit I will put within you. And I will remove the heart of stone from your flesh and give you a heart of flesh.
Ezekiel 36:26 (ESV)

Imagine the scene: a hot and arid desert, the sun high and relentless. The year is 1942, and a group of British soldiers finds themselves lost in the unforgiving terrain of North Africa. The Battle of El Alamein is in full swing with British forces, under the command of General Bernard Montgomery, squaring off against the famed German Afrika Korps led by Field Marshal Erwin Rommel.

This band of British soldiers is stranded without water deep behind enemy lines. They have lost all communication with their command. Dehydrated, demoralized, and desperate, they face a choice that goes against every instinct they have as soldiers: surrender to the enemy, or perish in the desert.

With heavy hearts, they approach the enemy camp with hands in the air, fully expecting a swift and brutal end. But, to their surprise, they are met not with bullets, but with canteens of water and a place in the shade. The German soldiers, recognizing the desperate condition of their enemies, provide them with sustenance, treating them with unexpected dignity and respect.

This moment, in the midst of a brutal and unforgiving war, displayed a surprising turn from expectations. The British soldiers turned away from their mission, their training, and their sworn duty in order to survive. And the German soldiers turned from their orders and their conditioning to show mercy.

Without making assumptions about the spiritual condition of the soldiers—after all, the Nazi regime was a force of great evil and their sins cannot be minimized—I share this story to illustrate the nature of the word "repentance." Each group of soldiers, in this instance, detoured from a path marked by death to one characterized by mercy.

In the wilderness of addiction, we often find ourselves stranded, lost, and desperately needing to make a similar choice. We need to lay down our arms, surrender our pride, our self-sufficiency, and our rebellion against God. This is the essence of repentance, which is *a turning away from ourselves and our sinful desires, and a turning toward the mercy and grace of God.*

The biblical definition of repentance is not simply about saying 'sorry' or feeling guilty about our sins. It is about changing course and setting a new path toward Jesus. It's about death and resurrection, about a transformation that starts within us and seeps into our actions. In other words, repentance

DAY 1 - REPENTANCE IS AN INVITATION

is not a stand-alone act. It isn't a solitary moment of regret or a fleeting wave of sorrow. Rather, it's the beginning of a journey toward something good, true, and life-giving.

When we repent, we lay down our old self, with all its insecurities, egoism, and false loves, and bury it in the grave. We part ways with the sin that clings so tightly, like shedding an old skin, and embrace the promise of a new life in Christ. We turn from the allure of a heart of stone, and look instead to the promise of a heart of flesh, as God assures us through Ezekiel:

> And I will give you a new heart, and a new spirit I will put within you. And I will remove the heart of stone from your flesh and give you a heart of flesh. (Ezekiel 36:26 ESV)

Thomas Watson rightly pointed out, "The two great graces essential to a saint in this life, are *faith* and *repentance.* These are the two wings by which he flies to heaven." [4] So, to repent is to receive grace, a gift from God, that works hand-in-hand with faith. It's more about realizing the vastness of God's mercy and love. Ray Ortlund encapsulates it beautifully when he says, "We have zero motivation to repent unless we see the mercy of God awaiting us. Not the slap of God, but the embrace of God." [5]

In the light of God's grace, repentance is an invitation. It's a chance to let go of the past, to be freed from the shackles

---

[4] Thomas Watson, *The Doctrine of Repentance* (1668; revised edition, e.g., Grand Rapids: Reformation Heritage Books, 2003).

[5] Ray Ortlund, "What Is True Repentance," *The Gospel Coalition*, December 5, 2012, https://www.thegospelcoalition.org/blogs/ray-ortlund/what-is-true-repentance/.

of sin, and to be reborn into a new life of love, hope, and peace. This new life is a God-fashioned life, one where our innermost desires and outward behaviors reflect the character of God Himself. And in this life, we discover the unending and unsurpassable grace of God that awaits us as we turn from our sinful ways toward His loving embrace.

* * *

Write Your Thoughts

- How can we regularly focus on seeking God's forgiveness instead of focusing on regret? What practical actions can we take every day to make this shift in our attitude?

- How does the story of the soldiers embody the essence of repentance? To better understand the power of mercy and grace, how could this play out in your own life?

- We understand that repentance is an ongoing process, not just a one-time action. How can this understanding help us or encourage us when we are struggling with long-standing habits or behaviors that dishonor God?

Create a New Rhythm

Whenever you are tempted to dwell in regret or guilt, remember that God is inviting you to dwell in Him and his forgiveness instead. He promises to give us a new heart if we repent and surrender to him. Pray and ask for his help to strengthen you as you turn away from your sin.

10

Day 2 - Rhythms of Repentance

...if you confess with your mouth that Jesus is Lord and believe in your heart that God raised him from the dead, you will be saved. For with the heart one believes and is justified, and with the mouth one confesses and is saved.
Romans 10:9-10 (ESV)

Eustace Scrubb, a skeptical and argumentative boy, is swept into the magical world of Narnia in C.S. Lewis's book, *The Voyage of the Dawn Treader*. During his journey, Eustace gives into his greed and steals from a dragon's hoard. As a result, he is transformed into a dragon, mirroring his inner state of greed and selfishness. This dramatic transformation prompts Eustace to realize how difficult and selfish he has been, spurring a profound sense of remorse and a desire for change.

In his quest to regain his human shape, Eustace meets Aslan, a character representing Christ in the Narnia series. Aslan

DAY 2 - RHYTHMS OF REPENTANCE

guides Eustace to strip away his dragon skin, which symbolizes repentance and transformation. Yet despite Eustace's earnest efforts, he finds himself unable to rid himself of the dragon skin on his own, symbolizing the impossibility of achieving personal redemption without God's help.

When Eustice finally surrenders and accepts the help of Aslan, this is how he describes the experience:

> The very first tear he made was so deep that I thought it had gone right into my heart. And when he began pulling the skin off, it hurt worse than anything I've ever felt. The only thing that made me able to bear it was just the pleasure of feeling the stuff peel off. You know - if you've ever picked the scab off a sore place. It hurts like billy-oh but it is such fun to see it coming away. [6]

After Aslan has torn away Eustace's dragon skin he throws him into a pool. Eustace emerges as a boy once again but he's changed fundamentally. The arrogant, self-centered boy is replaced by someone humbler and kinder, marking the start of his ongoing transformation. This transformative encounter with Aslan profoundly impacts Eustace's character, setting him on a new path for his life journey.

Just as true repentance is not something Eustace could do on his own, neither is our repentance simply an outward act of confession or making amends. Repentance is a deep-seated

---

[6] C.S. Lewis and Pauline Baynes, *The Voyage of the Dawn Treader: Full Color Collectors Edition* (New York: HarperTrophy, 2000), 108–109.

grace of God's Spirit that transforms the heart of a sinner from the inside out. It is spiritual medicine for the souls of those who follow Christ. It is an understanding of who we are, and more importantly, who God is.

When I come to the Lord in repentance, what helps me most is the image from Isaiah 64:8 (*ESV*):

> O LORD, you are our Father; we are the clay, and you are our potter; we are all the work of your hand.

In many ways, great and small, I try to be the potter of my life. I try to shape the clay of myself with my own strength and understanding, and I try to do the same with the clay of those around me. When I turn to God, I confess this to him.

The image of the potter and clay helps me to see how foolish my efforts have been and how misshapen I have made the clay. When I think about it this way, I find that I can gladly give the clay of myself over to the potter and be thankful; he is glad too, for this is how he has made things. It is right and good for the creature to submit to the hands of their creator, the potter, the one meant to shape the clay.

This is repentance. As the clay, this is my heartfelt prayer:

> God, I am in your hands. I am at your mercy. I give you my sin, my foolishness, my ignorance, my weakness, my talents, my wisdom, my strength, all of me. I am wholly dependent upon you to cleanse me of my sin and to shape me into who you want me to be.

While God does the heart work that allows us to come to Him, repentance means responding to his transformative power with

DAY 2 - RHYTHMS OF REPENTANCE

our own actions. Repentance often means *removing yourself* from people, places, and things that will draw you back into sin. This action feels sacrificial, but repentance is dying to our own efforts of trying to satisfy ourselves. It is dying to the part of us that is competing against fully trusting God. Repentance is finding your treasure in God.

For where your treasure is, there your heart will be also.
Matthew 6:21 (ESV)

* * *

Write Your Thoughts

- Drawing from Eustace's transformation, how can we apply the concept of "shedding our dragon skin" in practical terms in our recovery?

- In recovery, separation from environments or influences that encourage our addictive behavior is often necessary. How does this idea relate to "dying to our own efforts" as described in the passage?

- Share a practical example of "dying to our efforts" that could help someone in their recovery journey.

Create a New Rhythm

Spend five minutes in prayer to confess your sins to God. Then *take action to cut off any avenues of temptation* that would bring you back to that sin. Finally, rejoice in the fact that you are forgiven and free.

Make this routine a regular practice and experience the freedom that comes from casting your burdens on Jesus.

11

Day 3 - Repentance & Rest for Your Soul

"Are you tired? Worn out? Burned out on religion? Come to me. Get away with me and you'll recover your life. I'll show you how to take a real rest. Walk with me and work with me—watch how I do it. Learn the unforced rhythms of grace. I won't lay anything heavy or ill-fitting on you. Keep company with me and you'll learn to live freely and lightly."
Matthew 11:28-30 (MSG)

We are all prone to wandering down the wrong path. Thankfully, that's when we hear the gentle voice of Jesus calling us to "Come to me."

Repentance is the act of continually coming to Jesus. In Matthew 11:28-30, Jesus offers himself as the source of rest and relief for those who are weary from the struggles of life, including the burden of sin. By taking on His yoke and learning from Him, we can find rest for our souls and live freely and lightly. In other words, repentance involves surrendering ourselves to Jesus and allowing Him to lead and guide our lives, which leads to true and lasting peace.

If you have spent time in the recovery world, there is a good chance that you have heard about the 12 Steps of Alcoholics Anonymous (AA). They are a set of principles and actions that are designed to help people overcome alcoholism. Step 2 of AA says, "We came to believe that a Power greater than ourselves could restore us to sanity." There is only one true hope that can save us. The power that is greater than ourselves, the true "Higher Power," is the God described in the Bible. Any other "higher power" will prove to be neither high nor powerful.

Step 2 emphasizes realizing that there is a power greater than ourselves and that one cannot overcome this struggle alone. *We can't depend on our own strength and understanding but must depend on God, the higher power, to free us from our bondage.*

Step 5 requires individuals to admit to God, to themselves, and to another human being the exact nature of their wrongs. This step emphasizes the importance of taking responsibility for one's actions, acknowledging the harm they caused, and seeking forgiveness from God and others. The foundation of step 5 is *repentance* to God.

Step 7 involves humbly asking God to remove one's shortcomings. This step emphasizes the importance of acknowledging one's faults and seeking help from God to overcome them. Steps 7 and 10 meld together to create a healthy *rhythm of repentance* to God.

Step 10 requires individuals to continue to take personal inventory and promptly admit when they are wrong. This step emphasizes the importance of *ongoing self-reflection and repentance.*

When appropriately viewed through the lens of the Gospel, the 12 Steps promote repentance to the one true Higher Power. They rightly encourage us to recognize that our own strength and understanding are not enough, and will never be enough, to gain mastery over our sin and addictions. They encourage us to seek forgiveness and peace from God, take responsibility for our actions, and continue in self-reflection and repentance to God moving forward.

Here are some scriptures that correspond with the steps we have discussed:

- **Step 2:** Psalm 103:2-5 (*ESV*)

    Bless the Lord, O my soul, and forget not all his benefits, who forgives all your iniquity, who heals all your diseases, who redeems your life from the pit, who crowns you with steadfast love and mercy, who satisfies you with good so that your youth is renewed like the eagle's.

- **Step 5:** 1 John 1:7-9 (*ESV*)

    But if we walk in the light, as he is in the light, we have fellowship with one another, and the blood of Jesus his son cleanses us from all sin. If we say we have no sin, we deceive ourselves, and the truth is not in us. If we confess our sins, he is faithful and just to forgive us our sins and to cleanse us from all unrighteousness.

- **Step 7:** Galatians 5:22-25 (*ESV*)

    But the fruit of the spirit is love, joy, peace, patience, kind-

ness, goodness, faithfulness, gentleness, self-control; against such things there is no law. And those who belong to Christ Jesus have crucified the flesh with its passions and desires. If we live by the Spirit, let us also keep in step with the Spirit.

- **Step 10:** Psalm 139:23-24 (ESV)

Search me, O God, and know my heart! Try me and know my thoughts! And see if there be any grievous way in me, and lead me in the way everlasting!

* * *

Write Your Thoughts

- What is a yoke, and why does Jesus use the metaphor of a yoke in Matthew 11? (Google may be your friend here)

- Of the four steps from Alcoholics Anonymous discussed in this reading, which one seems the most challenging to you?

- What, according to the scriptures above, are the benefits of living in repentance?

Create a New Rhythm

Take five minutes to write down a brief list of those you may have wronged. Ask God to give you the courage to confide in someone trustworthy with this list and to make amends to those you need to make things right with.

12

Day 4 - A Repentance Letter

Have mercy on me, O God, according to your unfailing love; according to your great compassion blot out my transgressions.
Psalm 51:1 (NIV)

In Luke 15, Jesus tells the story of the Prodigal Son. In this story, a young man demands his inheritance from his father and goes off to waste it, living recklessly. This is an attack against his father and a mockery of his life and legacy. But when a famine hits the land, the young man is left with nothing. He realizes the error of his ways and decides to return home, repent, and ask for forgiveness.

As the wayward son comes to his senses, he says,

> I will arise and go to my father, and I will say to him, 'Father, I have sinned against heaven and before you. I am no longer worthy to be called your son. Treat

DAY 4 - A REPENTANCE LETTER

me as one of your hired servants.' And he arose and came to his father. But while he was still a long way off, his father saw him and felt compassion, and ran and embraced him and kissed him. (Luke 15:18-20 ESV)

What extravagant love the father showed the repentant son! Jesus' story illustrates the depth of a father's love and forgiveness. Despite his son's selfish actions and rebellion, the father never stopped loving him and was always eager to welcome him back with open arms.

This same unstoppable love applies to you and me. Our Heavenly Father is full of compassion and will abundantly pardon his children. Isaiah 55:7 says, "...let the wicked forsake his way, and the unrighteous man his thoughts; let him return to the Lord, that he may have compassion on him, and to our God, for he will abundantly pardon."

In Psalm 51, we read another story of repentance and grace. Like the prodigal son, King David rebelled and turned away from his Heavenly Father. He committed adultery with Bathsheba and had her husband, Uriah, killed to cover it up. When the prophet Nathan confronted David about his sin, David was overwhelmed with guilt and remorse.

David's sin was serious and harmful to himself and many others. Adultery and murder were punishable by death under the law of Moses, and those sins are only the most obvious of the many that David committed that year. After months of bottling it up, David finally turns to his Heavenly Father and opens the floodgates of his heart in a beautiful letter of repentance known to us as Psalm 51.

In this letter, adapted from the MSG version of Psalm 51, a

son or daughter is asking for forgiveness and repenting from self-centeredness, pride, and rebellion:

Dear Father,

Have mercy on me, not because of who I am, but because of who you are – because of your perfect, unrelenting love. My conscience is burdened with guilt and shame, and I can no longer bear it. I come before you, humbly and with a repentant heart, asking for your forgiveness.

Father, I know I have sinned against you in thought, word, and deed. But I also know that you are a God of mercy and compassion. You are slow to anger and abounding in unstoppable love, and you will not leave me.

I ask that you erase my wrong actions and then wash me clean. Create in me a clean heart, O God, and renew a right spirit within me. Forgive me, Father, and heal me of my sins.

You are a God of restoration and redemption. You can take my brokenness and turn it into something beautiful.

Thank you for your love and your grace. Thank you for your kindness; it has brought me to repentance. Thank you for being the kind of Father who never gives up on his children. I am sorry for what I have done, and I pray that you will forgive me and restore me.

DAY 4 - A REPENTANCE LETTER

I love you, Dad,

Your Child

* * *

Write Your Thoughts

- How was the famine in the parable of the Prodigal Son a good thing? What was the "famine" in your life that God used to bring you to repentance?

- How do you see your heavenly Father? Do you believe he sees you as the father in the parable sees his son?

- How has God received you with open arms when you have repented of your sin? If God forgave David of his very serious sin, why can't he forgive you?

Create a New Rhythm

Open your Bible to Psalm 51 and meditate on the words of David's letter to God. From now on, when you sin against God or someone else, try to pray some of the words of Psalm 51 to your Heavenly Father and rejoice in his forgiveness and freedom!

IV

Gratitude

*Day 1 - **What is Gratitude?***

*Day 2 - **Thanksgiving vs. Anxiety***

*Day 3 - **Locked Up & Thankful***

*Day 4 - **Entitlement: A "Screwtape" Letter***

13

Day 1 - What is Gratitude?

*Give thanks in all circumstances; for this is the will of
God
in Christ Jesus for you.*
1 Thessalonians 5:18 (ESV)

Gratitude is an attitude of appreciation, recognition, and thankfulness for something that has been received or experienced. It comes from realizing that everything in our lives is a gift.

Gratitude is also an act of the will. The default condition of the human heart is ingratitude. To develop a grateful heart, we must practice gratitude on a daily basis. When planted in abundance, gratitude will yield humility, dependence on God, and love for others.

Finally, gratitude is also a fundamental part of following Jesus. Consider the words of the apostle Paul that being grateful is "the will of God in Christ Jesus for you." It is God's will that we are thankful. Why? Because it is impossible to love God and truly worship him without being grateful to Him.

Consider this example of gratitude (my paraphrased version of Luke 17:11-19):

> One day, as Jesus was traveling, he came into a small village. By this point, his reputation had grown, so he was immediately recognized by ten lepers at the edge of town. Keeping their distance, as was the custom, so as not to spread their infection, the lepers shouted at Jesus. They begged him for mercy and asked him to heal them. (What faith they had!)
>
> Jesus simply responded, "Go and show yourselves to the priests." He had healed them instantly. But what happened next is shocking. As the ten lepers began running into town to show the priests that they were cleansed and able to rejoin society, *one of them stopped.* He turned back to Jesus and fell on the ground in gratitude. Jesus responded by asking the rhetorical question, "Where are the other nine that I healed?"
>
> Only one stayed to give thanks to God for this gift of healing.

As we are confronted with the reality of what God has done for us, our perspective shifts from self-centeredness to God-centeredness. We can't help but fall on the ground in gratitude at the feet of Jesus. Ultimately, gratitude is the only response to the greatest gift ever given: eternal salvation through Jesus Christ.

As we live in a state of gratitude, we are empowered to live a life of purpose, joy, and service to others. When we practice gratitude each day, we become immune to fear and resentment.

The choice is yours each morning when you rise: will you run through this life forgetting who cleansed you, *or* will you stop and give thanks?

> "Gratitude is the beginning of all virtues, and it is the first step towards heaven."
> – St. Augustine

* * *

Write Your Thoughts

- How would you define gratitude in your own words?

- What is different about "Christian gratitude" as opposed to ordinary gratitude?

- In what area of your life could you be more grateful to God? What is holding you back from being grateful in this area?

Create a New Rhythm

We must exhibit gratitude in our relationships with others. Find one person that you are grateful for and thank them today through a text message, phone call, or in-person conversation. Be specific in why you are thankful for them.

14

Day 2 - Thanksgiving vs. Anxiety

Do not be anxious about anything, but in everything by prayer and supplication with thanksgiving let your requests be made known to God.
Philippians 4:6 (ESV)

Corrie Ten Boom and her family were Dutch Christians imprisoned in a concentration camp during World War II for helping Jews escape the Nazis. Corrie and her sister, Betsie, began holding secret Bible studies in the concentration camp with the other prisoners. Although reading the Bible was not allowed within the camp, and they could be severely punished if caught, they kept studying the Bible together.

The women's barracks were shabby and completely infested with fleas. Corrie would grumble about the fleas, but Betsie always reminded her that they should give thanks in all circumstances, as the Bible teaches. Betsie quoted 1 Thessalonians 5:18, which says, "In *everything* give thanks, for this is the will of God in Christ Jesus concerning you."

Corrie was initially skeptical, but she agreed to give thanks for the fleas anyway. For months, the women led worship services in their barracks without being caught by the guards. It wasn't until later that Corrie learned that the fleas had been a disguised blessing. *The flea infestation had been the reason the guards would not enter their barracks and discover their Bible studies.* Yes, God uses even fleas for his glory!

The story of the fleas has become a powerful symbol of the importance of gratitude and the unexpected ways in which God can work in our lives. It is a testament to the faith and resilience of those who endured unimaginable suffering during the Holocaust and a reminder that even in the darkest circumstances, there is always something to be thankful for. As Betsie Ten Boom told her sister days before she died, "There is no pit so deep that He (God) is not deeper still." [7]

Martin Luther, one of the fathers of the protestant reformation, saw gratitude as a way of acknowledging our dependence on God and expressing our faith in His goodness and provision. He believed that gratitude is a powerful antidote to despair and anxiety. In one of his sermons, he wrote:

> When you are discouraged and full of doubt, when despair overwhelms you, call to mind the blessings of God and thank Him for them. This will strengthen your faith and give you the courage to face your troubles confidently.[8]

---

[7] Corrie ten Boom, *The Hiding Place* (Grand Rapids, MI: Chosen Books, 1971).

[8] Attributed to Martin Luther - exact source unknown. This quote may be a paraphrase rather than a direct quote.

DAY 2 - THANKSGIVING VS. ANXIETY

Thankfulness is the antivenom to the sting of anxiety that we all face in this life. Fear of death could have kept Corrie and Betsie from practicing their faith in the Nazi concentration camp, and it could have kept Martin Luther from standing on God's word in the face of militant opposition. Despite their anxiety, gratitude to God preserved their faith when all seemed lost. Be thankful to God in every circumstance; you may be surprised how your worries turn to gladness.

* * *

Write Your Thoughts

- What are the "fleas" in your life right now? What is that situation that you wish God would change?

- Take a moment to think about this: what reason could God have for not changing that circumstance right now? How could he be using it for your good and his glory?

- We all struggle with anxiety. List the top 3 things that you have been worrying over lately.

Create a New Rhythm

Take a moment to thank God for the "fleas" in your life. It seems ridiculous, but thank him for your blessings despite the hardship you are going through. From now on, every time you become anxious or fearful, say a prayer of thanksgiving to the God who is with you.

15

Day 3 - Locked Up & Thankful

Pray diligently. Stay alert, with your eyes wide open in gratitude. Don't forget to pray for us, that God will open doors for telling the mystery of Christ, even while I'm locked up in this jail. Pray that every time I open my mouth I'll be able to make Christ plain as day to them.
Colossians 4:2-4 (MSG)

During World War II, a Chinese Christian man was imprisoned in a concentration camp with other prisoners, including many other Christians. His job was to clean out the latrines. A "latrine" is an outdoor toilet with no plumbing; it is simply a hole dug into the ground to collect waste. Latrine duty was the worst job in the camp by far.

Despite the brutal and degrading nature of the work, he never complained. The other prisoners were amazed by his attitude and asked how he could remain positive in such terrible circumstances. He replied that he had chosen to focus on the good and to be thankful for every blessing, no matter how small. His fellow prisoners didn't understand. How could he be thankful for his blessings while given latrine duty in a WWII concentration camp? They asked him as much.

The imprisoned man responded, "While on latrine duty, the smell is so horrific that the guards stay far away, and I'm free to sing hymns and praise God without interruption." [9] This is a true heart of gratitude.

No matter your life's challenges, you have a reason to be grateful. Thankfulness doesn't imply that we ignore terrible things or try to make them better when possible. It means opening our perspective beyond the mess to something good. Because of Christ's grace and mercy, we are given a gift that surpasses all understanding. Even during our worst circumstances, we can find hope and joy in knowing *God is with us.*

But it's not just in hard times that we should give thanks. It's easy to forget about God's goodness and take our blessings for granted when things are going well. That's why we must cultivate a *rhythm* of gratitude, recognizing and appreciating all God has done for us.

Take a moment to thank our gracious God, who has blessed us beyond measure. And let's cultivate a heart of gratitude that overflows into every aspect of our lives, no matter how terrible they might seem.

* * *

Write Your Thoughts

---

[9] Adapted from a sermon illustration - author unknown.

- Picture a time when you were in a desperate situation, such as the Chinese man in the WWII concentration camp. What was your attitude during that time? Were you grateful or bitter?

- List ten things that you are grateful for.

Create a new Rhythm

Spend 5 minutes meditating on the passage below. Write it down on a note card or piece of paper and place it somewhere you will see daily as a reminder to be grateful to God.

> *Therefore let us be grateful for receiving a kingdom that cannot be shaken, and thus let us offer to God acceptable worship, with reverence and awe, for our God is a consuming fire.*
> Hebrews 12:28-29 (ESV)

16

Day 4 - Entitlement: A "Screwtape" Letter

Let all bitterness and wrath and anger and clamor and slander be put away from you, along with all malice. Be kind to one another, tenderhearted, forgiving one another, as God in Christ forgave you.
Ephesians 4:31-32 (ESV)

The Screwtape Letters is a novel by C.S. Lewis in which a senior demon named Screwtape writes letters to his nephew, Wormwood, a junior tempter, advising him how to lead humans away from God and towards sin and death.

The letter below is my version of a "Screwtape Letter." It, too, is written from the perspective of Screwtape coaching his nephew, Wormwood, in tactics to lead his human away from Christ.

One of his favorite tactics is the temptation of entitlement, which is the belief that we are inherently deserving of privileges

DAY 4 - ENTITLEMENT: A "SCREWTAPE" LETTER

or special treatment.

And don't forget, the perspective of the letter is from the demon's point of view, which is why when he talks about the "Enemy," he is referring to God.

> My Dear Wormwood,
>
> I commend you on your recent successes in tempting your human charge to indulge in entitlement that led them to fall back into addiction. Ah, entitlement, that most delightful poison! It is a potent weapon in turning humans away from God and is indeed the opposite of gratitude, the most revolting and powerful virtue.
>
> You see, Wormwood, gratitude is a terrifying thing. It leads humans to look outside of themselves, acknowledge the goodness in their lives, and give credit to their Creator. Gratitude shatters pride, the most beloved of sins.
>
> But entitlement, oh, how it feeds the ego! Entitlement is the glue that will hold them in their addiction or drive them to relapse. We must whisper in their ear that they are entitled to more, that others have wronged them, and that the world is cruel and unfair. This turns their gaze inward toward their perceived injustices and away from the blessings surrounding them.
>
> Entitlement (paired with addiction) is a fire that consumes from within, burning away any sense of

gratitude and leaving only bitterness, envy, and resentment in its wake. It is a tool we demons can use with great effect, as it blinds humans to the goodness in their lives and turns their hearts away from the Source of all goodness.

So, my dear Wormwood, keep up your excellent work. Tempt your charge to dwell on the slights they have suffered, to nurse their grievances, and to cultivate that most delicious of sins, entitlement. In doing so, you will ensure that gratitude, the most dangerous of virtues, will never take root in their hearts.

Your affectionate uncle,

Screwtape

* * *

Write Your Thoughts

- Can you identify instances in your life where you may have allowed entitlement to overshadow gratitude?

DAY 4 - ENTITLEMENT: A "SCREWTAPE" LETTER

- In the letter, Screwtape mentions that entitlement can lead us to relapse. How has entitlement played a role in your own addiction?

- The concept of entitlement is linked with resentment, a powerful force that can justify harmful actions. Can you think of situations where you or someone else justified negative behavior through a sense of entitlement or resentment? How might cultivating gratitude change the outcome of such situations?

Create a New Rhythm

In the Lord's prayer, Jesus modeled how we are to pray. One of the things he prayed for was deliverance from the evil one. Keeping the above "Screwtape" letter in mind, pray for God's protection from the evil one and his deliverance from temptation. Make this prayer a regular part of your routine, and ask a friend or pastor to pray it for you.

V

Forgiveness

Day 1 - **The Waterfall of Forgiveness**

Day 2 - **Extending Forgiveness**

Day 3 - **The Cost and Power of Forgiveness**

Day 4 - **Revenge: A "Screwtape" Letter**

17

Day 1 - The Waterfall of Forgiveness

He is so rich in kindness and grace that he purchased our
freedom
with the blood of his Son and forgave our sins.
Ephesians 1:7 (NLT)

Imagine yourself hopping on a series of large rocks in the middle of a mountain stream. As you move upstream from rock to rock, the sound of the birds and the wind in the trees is gradually drowned out by a continuous roar. You make your way around a bend in the stream, and before you is a magnificent waterfall. The water flows down the falls without stopping. Towering rock formations surround its edges, embracing the cascade. As the water enters the pool below, it churns and dances. A perpetual spray from the rocks at the falls' base mists the moss and ferns that frame the waterfall like a robe. The powerful waters shape and mold the riverbed as they pummel and smooth the rocks below.

God's forgiveness is a lot like this waterfall. Each droplet – every stream of water – represents God's grace and mercy revealed in His forgiveness. If you have ever felt a rock that is in the direct flow of the water coming off of a well-established waterfall, you know how smooth and round the rock has become. In the same way, God gradually softens the hard, unyielding stone of our hearts, smoothing out its imperfections and reshaping it over time. God's forgiveness is powerful. His forgiveness is transformational.

Consider also how the waterfall purifies. The transformation brought on by the cascade is one of purification and cleansing. As the water rushes down, it carries away the dirt and the rubble collected along the path, just as God's forgiveness purifies us and washes away our sins and our guilt.

Finally, imagine a quiet pool of deep water further downstream from the cleansing falls. It is like a mirror, calm and tranquil. This mirror pool reflects the sun's glory just as our lives, touched by forgiveness, reflect God's love.

Have you ever stopped to ask *why* God would forgive you? I can tell you, this forgiveness did not come cheap. In Ephesians 1:7, Paul gives us the answer. We are forgiven, 1) through his blood, 2) because of the riches of his grace.

Jesus paid the ultimate price by laying down his life and drinking the entire cup of God's wrath for you. The forgiveness of your sins cost him everything. There never has been – nor will there ever be – a greater love than this.

So what now? What are we to do now that we have experienced God's forgiveness? Further on in Ephesians, Paul has another answer for us: "Be kind to one another, tenderhearted, forgiving one another, as God in Christ forgave you" (Ephesians 4:32). Embrace the call to forgive as we have been forgiven. Just as God, through Christ, reconciled us to Himself by his blood, let us extend forgiveness to those who have wronged us. For in forgiveness, we reflect the heart of our Heavenly Father and open the door to healing and restoration.

If you have not experienced God's forgiveness, this is your invitation. The loving Creator and Ruler of all things, the God that sent His son so that His forgiveness might be offered to you, invites you to come to him.

In him we have redemption through his blood, the forgiveness of our trespasses, according to the riches of his grace.
Ephesians 1:7 (ESV)

* * *

Write Your Thoughts

- How does the metaphor of the waterfall embody the idea of God's forgiveness? Can you think of other metaphors for his forgiveness?

- In what ways does God's forgiveness transform and purify us? Can you share a personal experience when forgiveness brought about transformation or purification?

- Ephesians 4:32 suggests that we should extend forgiveness as we have been forgiven by God. How do you see this call to action playing out in your life? Are there specific challenges or opportunities related to this?

- The final paragraph extends an invitation to experience God's forgiveness. Have you experienced God's forgiveness? If you have not, what obstacles are in your way?

Create a New Rhythm

Every human being that will ever live is faced with the same reality: we stand rightly condemned before a just God in need of a savior's forgiveness – a forgiveness that we do not deserve and cannot earn. God's forgiveness is freely offered to you. Today and *every day,* cry out to Jesus and embrace the forgiveness that he won for you with his blood.

> *Whoever believes in the Son has eternal life; whoever does not obey the Son shall not see life, but the wrath of God remains on him.*
> John 3:36 (ESV)

18

Day 2 - Extending Forgiveness

He does not deal with us according to our sins, nor repay us according to our iniquities. For as high as the heavens are above the earth, so great is his steadfast love toward those who fear him; as far as the east is from the west, so far does he remove our transgressions from us.
Psalm 103:10-12 (ESV)

Think of a time when someone really wronged you. Maybe they spread harmful lies about you, stole from you, or even abused you.

Painful moments like these can make reconciliation and healing seem impossible. Even if the person who hurts us is sorry, it can feel like there is no way to get past it. And yet, we are called to forgive. Matthew 6:14-15 (ESV) says, "For if you forgive others their trespasses, your heavenly Father will also forgive you, but if you do not forgive others their trespasses, neither will your Father forgive your trespasses." Forgiveness is an act of obedience that brings *healing and restoration* not only to our relationships but also to our own souls.

It is important to recognize that the call to forgiveness *does not negate or diminish the pain* caused by the wrongdoing. Consider the profound act of forgiveness displayed by the families of the victims of the Charleston church shooting of 2015. Forgiving the shooter did not make their pain and loss go away. The sorrow that filled the hearts of the families who lost their loved ones in the Charleston church shooting, including their pastor, Clementa C. Pinckney, is unimaginable. Yet, in the face of this immense tragedy, these families made a choice that defied human understanding. They followed Jesus and embraced forgiveness as their response instead of revenge.

The secular world could not understand why the victims' families offered forgiveness to the murderer of their loved ones, but Scripture tells us why. *Those Christians were able to forgive because they knew that they had been forgiven.* Psalm 103:10 (ESV) says, "He does not deal with us according to our sins, nor repay us according to our iniquities." Instead, he pardons our sins because of the blood of his son, Jesus Christ.

In the face of the tragic killing, how could they forgive? Because they had experienced the transforming forgiveness of their savior. Experiencing ultimate forgiveness from God enabled them to forgive.

The transformative power of forgiveness extends to each one of us. When we choose forgiveness, we embrace a path that leads to healing, restoration, and reconciliation. Forgiveness is not a sign of weakness; it is an act of obedience to God that acknowledges the massive debt that we ourselves have been forgiven.

DAY 2 - EXTENDING FORGIVENESS

* * *

Write Your Thoughts

- Reflect on Matthew 6:14-15. How does this passage challenge your understanding of forgiveness? What is the connection between receiving forgiveness yourself and extending forgiveness to others?

- Think about the transformative power of forgiveness in your own life. Can you recall a time when extending or receiving forgiveness brought about healing and reconciliation?

- Are there hurts, grievances, or grudges that you have been holding onto? What impact have these had on your life and relationships? Jesus forgave those who crucified Him— how might His ultimate act of forgiveness encourage you to forgive someone in your life?

Create a New Rhythm

Take time to pray this prayer to the Lord:

> *Gracious Heavenly Father, I humbly come before you, acknowledging the depth of my need for your forgiveness and grace. Remove my bitterness and resentment and fill my heart with your love and compassion. Help me to forgive those who have wronged me, just as you have forgiven me. Yours is the glory. Amen.*

19

Day 3 - The Cost and Power of Forgiveness

...bearing with one another and, if one has a complaint against another, forgiving each other; as the Lord has forgiven you, so you also must forgive. And above all these put on love, which binds everything together in perfect harmony.
Colossians 3:13-14 (ESV)

Joseph, the favored son of Jacob, faced deep betrayal and hardship at the hands of his brothers. They sold him into slavery, tore him away from his family, and left him to navigate the treacherous path of Egyptian servitude. Through the twists and turns of his life, Joseph eventually rose to a position of great authority in Pharaoh's court.

Years later, Joseph had a remarkable encounter with his brothers. They came to Egypt seeking help during a severe famine. Unknown to them, it was Joseph whom they appeared before to ask for aid. Instead of harboring resentment and seeking revenge, Joseph chose the path of forgiveness. He did not treat them as their sins had deserved. He wept openly, embraced his brothers, and declared, "Do not be distressed or angry with yourselves because you sold me here, for God sent me before you to preserve life" (Genesis 45:5 ESV). Later, he has this to say: "You meant evil against me, but God meant it for good, to bring it about that many people should be kept alive, as they are today" (Genesis 50:20 ESV).

Joseph's journey of forgiveness highlights the remarkable transformation that occurs when we choose to release bitterness and extend grace. Instead of seeking retribution, he recognized God's sovereign plan at work. He acknowledged that what his brothers meant for evil, God used for good. Joseph's forgiveness led to reconciliation, restoration, and the preservation of his family.

Forgiveness comes at a cost. Joseph had every reason to hold onto resentment and seek revenge. Maintaining our grudge toward those who hurt us can seem valuable to us. We may feel like we need to hold onto it to maintain control and protect ourselves from further harm. But this kind of "power" only brings destruction and ultimately death. Joseph chose to let go of those things and bear the pain of his brothers' betrayal by extending forgiveness. He released them from the burden of guilt and chose a path of healing and reconciliation instead.

Joseph's forgiveness is a small example of God's forgiveness for those he saves in Christ. When we choose to forgive, we mirror the forgiveness we have received from our Heavenly Father. By reflecting Christ, we shine hope, life, and light into the lives of those around us.

DAY 3 - THE COST AND POWER OF FORGIVENESS

* * *

Write Your Thoughts

- Joseph's response to his brothers was marked by grace and reconciliation, even after enduring years of betrayal and hardship. How did Joseph's perspective on God's sovereignty over the painful events in his life influence his ability to forgive? How can you apply this perspective in your own life?

- Forgiveness often involves bearing with one another and releasing our grievances against one another. In light of Joseph's story, what practical steps can we take to bear with one another and extend forgiveness, even when it is challenging or undeserved?

- Reflecting on Joseph's statement to his brothers in Genesis 50:20 (see above), how can we embrace the perspective that God can use even the most painful experiences for a greater purpose? How can this perspective shape our willingness to forgive and trust in God's sovereignty?

Create a New Rhythm

What is the main barrier that keeps you from forgiving that one person you just can't seem to forgive? Ask God to break down these barriers in your heart and give you grace to forgive.

20

Day 4 - Revenge: A "Screwtape" Letter

Let all bitterness and wrath and anger and clamor and slander be put away from you, along with all malice. Be kind to one another, tenderhearted, forgiving one another, as God in Christ forgave you.
Ephesians 4:31-32 (ESV)

Let's rephrase this verse from the perspective of C.S. Lewis' fictional demon "Screwtape." Here's what the demon might say to you about the ideas expressed in Ephesians 4:31-32:

"Hold fast to all bitterness and wrath and anger and clamor and slander, along with all malice. Be harsh to one another, hard-hearted, refusing to forgive one another, as if you were not forgiven by God in Christ."

Recall that *The Screwtape Letters* is a novel written by C.S. Lewis in which a senior demon named "Screwtape" writes letters to his nephew "Wormwood", who is a junior tempter, advising him on how to lead humans away from God and towards sin and death.[10]

Here's another of our versions of a "Screwtape Letter." It, too, is written from the perspective of Screwtape coaching his nephew, Wormwood, in tactics to lead humans away from Christ. When the below passage talks about the "Enemy," it is referring to God. Remember, this letter is from the demon's point of view:

> My Dear Wormwood,
>
> I note with some concern your recent report on the spiritual status of your patient. It appears that the Enemy's agent is making headway with that most troublesome of practices: forgiveness. This could be a serious setback for us if not countered appropriately and swiftly.
>
> Remember, dear Wormwood, forgiveness is the Enemy's masterstroke, a diabolical plot of unconditional love and absurd benevolence. It's a weapon that disarms us, rendering our best tactics of condemnation, judgment, and revenge utterly futile. Our power rests in the human ability to hold grudges, to seek revenge, and to judge harshly, not this nonsensical notion of forgiveness.
>
> Your patient must come to believe that condemnation and bitterness are the just responses to wrongs done unto him. Encourage him to perceive every slight – every single offense – as a personal affront that must be avenged. Let him believe that it is not

---

[10] C.S. Lewis, *The Screwtape Letters* (New York: HarperCollins, 2001).

only his right but his duty to resent the ones who have wronged him. The sweetness of revenge must be his most desired dessert, and he must crave the delicious satisfaction of vengeance.

You see, Wormwood, our advantage lies in the human tendency towards reciprocity. They are wired to return like for like, eye for an eye, tooth for a tooth. Play on this, and amplify it. His need to 'settle the score' must override any misguided notions of forgiveness the Enemy's agent might plant in his mind.

Moreover, it is crucial that the patient does not understand that forgiveness is an act of liberation for the forgiver. He must believe that by holding onto anger, resentment, and bitterness, he is in control. This should not be difficult. Humans are all too willing to create their own bonds. The fact that forgiveness would set your human free should never enter his mind.

And should the topic of forgiveness arise, there are several ways to turn it to our advantage. Convince him that it is a sign of weakness. Persuade him that it will only open him up to being hurt again. It is even in the enemy's book, but do not steer him there; it is too risky. If he insists on forgiving, then preserve a root of bitterness in his heart so that he never lets go of the offense.

Always remember, Wormwood, that our aim is not just to lead them away from the Enemy but also to distort their understanding of His teachings. Let them believe that their path of bitterness and revenge is the righteous one, and that forgiveness is nothing more than an impractical, foolish notion.

Your affectionate uncle,

Screwtape

* * *

Write Your Thoughts

- What does this letter say about the human inclination towards revenge rather than forgiveness? In what ways do you observe these tendencies in your own life?

- The demon writing the letter explains that humans should be convinced that forgiveness is a sign of weakness. How does this idea contradict the teachings of the Bible, particularly Ephesians 4:31-32 (see above)?

DAY 4 - REVENGE: A "SCREWTAPE" LETTER

- The letter suggests that one of the devil's tactics is to distort our understanding of God's teachings. In what ways might you have experienced or witnessed this distortion, specifically regarding the concepts of revenge and forgiveness?

Create a New Rhythm

Find two or three Bible passages that deal with forgiveness or revenge. Write these down on notecards or a sheet of paper and keep them in your car, nightstand, or anywhere that you can access easily. When Satan tempts you to take revenge and harbor bitterness toward someone else, pull out these verses and meditate on the truth of what God says.

VI

Spiritual Disciplines

Day 1 – **Spiritual Discipline**

Day 2 – **God's Word to Humanity**

Day 3 – **The Privilege of Prayer**

Day 4 – **Freedom to Worship**

21

Day 1 - Spiritual Discipline

Train yourself to be godly. For physical training is of some value, but godliness has value for all things, holding promise for both the present life and the life to come.
1 Timothy 4:7-8 (NIV)

What is a Spiritual Discipline? Spiritual disciplines are the practices or habits followers of Jesus engage in to deepen their relationship with God and become more like Christ. They are the means by which we cultivate godliness and build Christ-like character. When we practice these disciplines, we experience the joy and peace that come from a vibrant relationship with God.

The following are examples of spiritual disciplines:

Inward Disciplines:

- **Prayer** - Communicating with God, including praise, thanksgiving, confession, and requests.
- **Bible** - Reading, studying, meditating on, and memorizing Scripture.
- **Meditation** - Focusing your mind on God and His Word to increase understanding and apply it to life.
- **Worship** - expressing adoration, reverence, thanks, surrender, and praise through singing or other means of expression.

Outward Disciplines:

- **Service** - Serving others in the name of Christ, often through acts of kindness, charity, and justice.
- **Fellowship** - Building relationships with other believers for mutual encouragement, accountability, and growth.
- **Evangelism** - Sharing the good news of Jesus Christ with others.
- **Discipleship** - Intentionally encouraging others and sharing what God is teaching you.
- **Generosity/Stewardship** - Giving your resources (time, talent, and money) to support the work of God in the world.

In his first letter to the Corinthians, the Apostle Paul uses the analogy of a race to describe our spiritual journey. Just as athletes discipline their bodies and train rigorously to compete in a race, we must exercise spiritual discipline to run our spiritual race.

Here's what he says: "Do you not know that in a race all the runners run, but only one gets the prize? Run in such a way as to get the prize. Everyone who competes in the games goes into

DAY 1 - SPIRITUAL DISCIPLINE

strict training. They do it to get a crown that will not last, but we do it to get a crown that will last forever. Therefore, I do not run like someone running aimlessly; I do not fight like a boxer beating the air. No, I strike a blow to my body and make it my slave so that after I have preached to others, I myself will not be disqualified for the prize" (1 Corinthians 9:24-27 NIV).

Imagine if someone woke you up one morning and said you had ten minutes before the race began. You did not know about the race, you are not a runner, and you definitely haven't trained at all. How is this race going to go? Not very well. You will likely finish last place – if you finish at all – and be miserable the entire time.

For many of us, this is a summary of our spiritual life every day. We wake up unprepared for what is to come and stumble through trials and temptations like we are winging a math test. It doesn't have to be this way! If you are in Christ, he has won for you the ability to approach the throne of grace in prayer. He has secured for you the gift of the Holy Spirit, who helps you understand God's word. He invites you to join him by participating and serving in the church and giving generously.

But remember, as with any discipline, spiritual disciplines are not about being perfect, but about growing and maturing. Discipline is a process, and often reveals our weakness and need for God. Being aware of our need helps us to depend on him more and receive life from Him.

Spiritual disciplines are NOT for the purpose of earning favor with God or achieving salvation. Christ has already purchased salvation on the cross! Spiritual disciplines are our means of drawing nearer to God, learning more about him, and becoming more like him. They are for his glory and for our good.

As we seek to grow in our spiritual disciplines, let us remember that it is not by our strength but by the grace of God that we grow. "For 'In him we live and move and have our being'" (Acts 17:28 ESV). So let us run our race trusting in his love and promises to the glory of the King.

* * *

Write Your Thoughts

- Think about the analogy of running a race. Why is this significant when compared with our spiritual journey?

- List one or more spiritual disciplines that you currently practice (or want to start practicing). How can these practices help you deepen your relationship with God?

- Spiritual disciplines are not intended to earn God's love but to deepen our relationship with Him. How does this perspective shift your understanding of spiritual discipline?

- Write down what motivates you to engage in these practices. What is your primary goal in practicing spiritual discipline?

Create a New Rhythm

Being completely honest with yourself, write down how many times per week you engage in the following disciplines:

- Bible reading
- Intentional time in prayer
- Personal worship
- Corporate worship (gathered in worship with other believers at church)
- Fellowship with other believers (small group)
- Evangelism
- Discipleship
- Acts of charitable service for others

The purpose of this exercise is to get a baseline from which you and your mentor/group can begin encouraging each other to practice these more and track your growth in spiritual discipline.

22

Day 2 - God's Word to Humanity

> *God means what he says. What he says goes. His powerful Word is sharp as a surgeon's scalpel, cutting through everything, whether doubt or defense, laying us open to listen and obey. Nothing and no one can resist God's Word. We can't get away from it—no matter what.*
> Hebrews 4:12-13 (MSG)

The Bible is God's Holy Word to humanity. It is 1) Inspired, 2) Infallible, 3) Inerrant, 4) Authoritative, and 5) Sufficient.

An adequate explanation of these terms is outside the scope of this lesson. However, each of them is of vital importance, and I would encourage you to look up more about them on your own. Suffice it to say, "The law of the LORD is perfect, reviving the soul" (Psalm 19:7 ESV).

And because it is perfect and comes from a perfect God, it is trustworthy. Paul tells his little brother in the faith, Timothy, that "All Scripture is breathed out by God and profitable for teaching, for reproof, for correction, and for training in righteousness, that the man of God may be complete, equipped for every good work" (2 Timothy 3:16 ESV).

In his book *The Practice of Godliness*, Jerry Bridges identifies five methods of taking in God's Word: hearing, reading, studying, memorizing, and meditating.[11] We must engage in all of these to fully experience Scripture as God intends.

Here is an example of what each of these might look like in your weekly routine:

1. **Hearing** - Pay close attention to the sermon taught by a Bible-teaching pastor at church (Revelation 1:3).
2. **Reading** - Read your Bible every day. Go through one book of the Bible at a time and read from it every day until you have read it from beginning to end. Then pick another book and repeat until you have read the entire Bible. Then repeat! There are many great Bible reading plans you can use as well.
3. **Studying** - Write down your questions and observations as you read the Bible. Then use what God has given you to find the answers and dig deeper. These can include the footnotes of a study Bible, a commentary, or asking your pastor or a mature Christian. This is where most Christians falter. Studying takes time, and we often don't want to commit our time. But as a wise man once said, "You always find time for what is important to you." Reading gives us breadth, but study gives us depth. This

---

[11] Jerry Bridges, *The Practice of Godliness* (Colorado Springs, CO: NavPress, 1983).

is where the gold is found (Proverbs 2:1-5).
4. **Memorizing** - Choose a favorite verse or passage and memorize it. Write it on a note card and carry it with you. Read it throughout the day and practice saying it to a friend until you know it. Then do the same with another verse. You will be surprised how much this simple practice will change your heart (Psalm 119:11).
5. **Meditating** - "The word meditate, as used in the Old Testament, literally means to murmur or to mutter and, by implication, to talk to oneself. When we meditate on the Scriptures, we talk to ourselves about them, turning over in our minds the meanings, the implications, and the applications to our own lives." Studying is an academic activity, while meditating is an introspective and heavenward undertaking.

Let's address a few common pitfalls when it comes to reading the Bible.

First, *it's easy to get confused* or feel like we don't understand what we're reading. That's okay! The greatest Bible scholars in the world were confused the first time they read that passage, too. That's where a commitment to diligent study will increase your understanding. As your understanding grows, your joy will grow exponentially.

Second, we can find *our minds wandering while we read* or even feel bored. This is because we don't understand what we're reading. The God of the universe is talking to you! As He grants you wisdom and understanding, you will find it impossible to be bored while reading His Word.

Finally, we can fall into *the trap of legalism*. This is where we read our Bibles simply to check a box or satisfy our sense of self-accomplishment. This is obedience for the wrong reason, and it does not please God. *The root of legalism is pride:* when I do well at reading my Bible, I relish in my accomplishment and what a good Christian I am. But when I miss a few days of Bible reading, I am depressed and defeated. When we live legalistically, we commit the sin of pride, and we also deprive ourselves of the joy of the salvation Jesus won for us. Rather than focusing on what you can do, try shifting your focus to what he has done for you, and rest in his grace.

Bottom line, we read the Bible to see Jesus. It's through His Word that God reveals His character, His will, His plan of salvation through Jesus Christ, and His guidance for living a life that brings him glory. By immersing ourselves in Scripture, our minds are renewed and our hearts filled with joy.

* * *

Write Your Thoughts

- Have you felt encouraged or discouraged by your Bible reading lately? If so, why? How might engaging in discussions about Scripture with other people in your life facilitate a deeper understanding and personal application of biblical truths?

- In what ways have you experienced the Bible's ability to "pierce" through your thoughts and intentions, revealing areas of your life in need of transformation?

- How does memorizing Scripture play a role in overcoming challenges and temptations in life?

Create a New Rhythm

Create your own personal Bible reading plan. This can include a reading plan you find online or one you design yourself. Schedule a time each day of the week to spend time in God's Word. Try to include all 5 methods of Scripture intake in some way during the week. Finally, share this plan with your mentor/group and ask them to do it with you if they don't have their own plan already. If you stick to your plan for 30 days, you will be a different person—I guarantee it.

23

Day 3 - The Privilege of Prayer

*And he said to them, 'When you pray, say: Father,
hallowed be your name. Your kingdom come. Give us
each day our daily bread, and forgive us our sins, for we
ourselves forgive everyone who is
indebted to us. And lead us not into temptation.*
Luke 11:204 (ESV)

Do you want to hear something sad? The most consistent season of prayer in my life was when I was wading through the madness of late addiction and stepping into the uncharted territory of early recovery. It's a disheartening truth because it took immense turmoil in my life to wake me up to the reality of my need for prayer. The truth is that I need prayer every day!

Here are truths I've learned about prayer:
   Prayer is our direct connection to God. - We can pray to the Father because of what Jesus has done on our behalf.

He laid down his life for us to make a way for us to be with him. Our prayers are heard because he still stands as our mediator to the Father. It is crucial that we understand this point because it means that we don't have to clean ourselves up before approaching God in prayer. We come before him with the spotless record of Jesus.

There are a variety of ways to structure our prayers. - There is no magic formula, but there are some helpful ideas. For example, you can use the Lord's Prayer as a blueprint or use the acronym A.C.T.S. (Adoration, Confession, Thanksgiving, Supplication). Praying the Scriptures is one of the best ways to pray. When you use a Scripture passage as your prayer guide it anchors your prayers in God's unchanging truth and aligns your requests with His will. The book of Psalms is a good place to start—just pick a Psalm and pray it back to the Lord.

Ultimately, our prayers should be natural and not forced. - Imagine if I only talked to my wife when I needed something from her. And when I asked, I always followed a scripted formula. That wouldn't go over well even the first time, much less if I did that every day for years! When we pray, we must feel free to approach the Lord in humility and authenticity.

Prayer ought to be a habit, but it is more than a habit. - It's a lifeline. It's a daily communion with the maker of all things. Think of it this way - just as any earthly relationship thrives on steady communication, our bond with God grows through regular dialogue. *Moreover, daily prayer aligns your will with His, nurtures your dependence on Him, and cultivates a heart of gratitude and trust.*

Remember, patience is key! - Our prayers may not be answered in the timeframe or manner we expect. Sometimes God's response is "not yet" or "no." He calls us to persist in prayer, placing our trust in His unmatched wisdom and perfect timing.

Lastly, there is power in the shared experience of prayer. - While our individual dialogues with God are precious, it is important to pray together with family, in small groups, or within the larger church community. Such shared prayers weave us together, fostering unity and mutual encouragement.

* * *

Write Your Thoughts

Reflect on the passages below and write down one takeaway from each passage:

- *Do not be anxious about anything, but in everything by prayer and supplication with thanksgiving let your requests be made known to God. And the peace of God, which surpasses all understanding, will guard your hearts and your minds in Christ Jesus. (Philippians 4:6-7 ESV)*

- *Rejoice always, pray without ceasing, give thanks in all circumstances; for this is the will of God in Christ Jesus for you. (1 Thessalonians 5:16-18 ESV)*

- *Therefore, confess your sins to one another and pray for one another, that you may be healed. The prayer of a righteous person has great power as it is working. (James 5:16 ESV)*

- *King David composed this psalm as a result of Nathan the prophet convicting him of his sins, both in his committing adultery with Bathsheba and in his arranging for the murder of Bathsheba's husband, Uriah. This is King David's appeal to God's gracious character as the grounds for his cry for forgiveness. (Psalm 51)*

Create a New Rhythm

Write down some specific times of the day that you could intentionally pray. For example, this could be when you first wake up in the morning, when you are driving to work, or during the last five minutes of your lunch break. Create the habit of praying *throughout the day* to experience a constant connection with your Savior.

24

Day 4 - Freedom to Worship

*I appeal to you therefore, brothers, by the mercies of
God, to present your bodies as a living sacrifice, holy and
acceptable to God,
which is your spiritual worship.*
Romans 12:1 (ESV)

Imagine a metronome, a simple instrument that marks a steady rhythm for musicians. Now envision this metronome as the steady beat of our life in Christ—an unending rhythm of worship that marches in step with the grace of God.

But this rhythm isn't exclusive to the echoes of Sunday worship services. It pulses in every heartbeat, in every moment of our daily life. When we're praying, reading God's Word, working, building relationships, even in our times of rest, this beat serves as a constant reminder to sync our lives to the rhythm of God.

Just like the metronome sets the tempo for the musicians,

God sets the tempo for our lives. We aren't the composers but rather the instruments skillfully directed by God in His grand symphony.

What exactly is worship? Worship is the act and attitude of giving praise and adoration. We all worship. We can't help it. This is how God made us. And often, we worship the creation rather than the Creator. But God is the only one *worthy* of our worship.

When an Olympic gymnast wins the gold medal, she is rightly honored for her achievement. It would be wrong to put the gymnast who came in last place on the first-place podium and present her with the gold medal. Only the winner is *worthy* of that honor.

Revelation 5 might be the most stunning passage in all of Scripture. We find ourselves in the throne room of the living God, surrounded by his angels who proclaim his praise continually. The apostle John, who is narrating this scene, is weeping because no one can be found who is worthy to open the scroll with seven seals. John writes in Revelation 5:5, 12 (ESV):

> And one of the elders said to me, "Weep no more; behold, the Lion of the tribe of Judah, the Root of David, has conquered, so that he can open the scroll and its seven seals… worthy is the Lamb who was slain, to receive power and wealth and wisdom and might and honor and glory and blessing."

Worship is not just a Sunday event. It is a part of everything we do. It involves a consistent recognition of His majesty. We should worship in our commonplace moments, the ones filled with everyday chores and casual conversations—as well as during our extraordinary moments filled with celebrations, challenges, and transformative experiences. In all these, we are called to live our lives as an act of worship.

Our worship culminates every Lord's Day when we gather together as a church to worship the King of Kings through corporate worship, the preaching of the Word, and fellowship with one another.

The writer of Hebrews says, "And let us consider how to stir up one another to love and good works, not neglecting to meet together, as is the habit of some, but encouraging one another, and all the more as you see the Day drawing near."[12]

It is a privilege to worship God. In the grand symphony of God's story, may every note and beat of our lives sing a song of worship, resounding with the recognition and celebration of God's supreme worth.

* * *

Write Your Thoughts

- How does the image of a metronome, keeping a steady beat, relate to your understanding of worship as a daily rhythm?

- How do you incorporate worship into your everyday life

---

[12] Hebrews 10:24–25 (English Standard Version).

beyond traditional Sunday services or prayer times? Are there areas in your life where you find it challenging to integrate worship?

- How do you experience personal worship, and how does it differ from your experience of communal worship? How do both contribute to your spiritual growth?

- How can you transform your work, leisure activities, relationships, and even rest into acts of worship? Be specific.

Create a New Rhythm

We sometimes think of going to church on Sunday as a drudge. Not anymore! The most powerful way to transform your worship is to change how you think about it. Adopt this new way of thinking and structure your week accordingly:
New mindset:
1) *I can worship God in everything I do by seeking to do it in a*

way that honors him.

2) *Sunday morning worship is the highlight of my week, and everything else is building toward it.*

Some ways that my life might reflect this:

- I find out what Biblical text will be preached on Sunday and read it on Saturday in preparation.
- I go to bed early Saturday night to be rested (Saturday Night Live = Sunday Morning Dead!)
- I invite others to church with me so that they can share in my joy.

VII

Peace & Patience

Day 1 - **Shalom in the Hurricane**

Day 2 - **Practicing Peace**

Day 3 - **Active Patience**

Day 4 - **Patience: A "Screwtape" Letter**

25

Day 1 - Shalom in the Hurricane

Do not be anxious about anything, but in every situation, by prayer and petition, with thanksgiving, present your requests to God. And the peace of God, which transcends all understanding, will guard your hearts and your minds in Christ Jesus.
Philippians 4:6-7 (ESV)

Have you ever been inside a hurricane? Hurricanes are powerful and chaotic forces of destruction, but at the center of a hurricane is an eye of calm. I would never want to be in a hurricane, but if I had to be in one, the eye would be the best place to be. A hurricane symbolizes the turmoil of this world—a storm of conflict, fear, and suffering that causes chaos and destruction. In the eye of the storm, we can find the peace of God. Though the winds whirl around us, within the eye, there is calm and peace.

The peace of God transcends all understanding and is unchanging despite life's hurricanes. This peace, like the eye of the storm, doesn't whisk us out of the hurricane, but provides us with stability and clarity in the midst of chaos. As we remain in the eye of the peace of God, we rest in the assurance of His presence, His goodness, and His control over all things. This divine peace serves as our refuge through life's fiercest storms. We all yearn for respite from worry, anxiety, and strife. The world gives promises of peace. It offers many comforts and provides an escape from the chaos. But there is a significant difference between the false and fleeting peace the world offers and the enduring peace God provides.

In Hebrew, God's peace is known as "Shalom." Shalom denotes much more than an absence of conflict. It embodies a sense of wholeness and completeness, and it is a reflection of God's own character. Shalom is found in Christian community. It is the divine harmony of hearts attuned to God and His Kingdom work, together trusting in His faithfulness, obeying His commands, and resting in His love.

In the Philippians 4 passage above, we see that the peace of God is a gift given to us. It is not something we can earn. We simply receive the peace of God in faith. Yet, in the same passage, Paul instructs us on how to order our lives to receive the peace of God in faith.

So how do we trust God and open ourselves up to receive the peace he has for us? We do it by resisting anxious thoughts and surrendering our "control" and our cares to God by praying, petitioning, and giving thanks to God. In other words, resting in God, depending on him, and giving thanks to God for all things is the key to experiencing his peace. He is good, and all things are from him and through him and belong to him. This is where the gift of peace is found. It is at the feet of the almighty God who calls us his beloved.

As followers of Jesus, we are called to reflect God's peace to those around us. This is how we participate with Jesus in bringing his shalom to the world. As God's ambassadors, we are to carry his peace with us in every aspect of life, and that begins with sharing the good news of the Gospel of Jesus Christ. In every situation, may we present our requests to God, with thanksgiving, letting His peace, which transcends all understanding, guard our hearts and minds in Christ Jesus. May we face the hurricanes of life not with fear, but with the steadfast assurance of His power and his peace.

* * *

Write Your Thoughts

- Today's reading uses the metaphor of the eye of a hurricane to represent the peace of God. How does this imagery resonate with your personal experiences of peace during hard times?

- Think about the fleeting peace offered by the world vs. the enduring peace provided by God. Can you share a personal example of how you experienced this contrast? How did the peace of God make a difference in that situation?

- How does the Hebrew concept of "Shalom" redefine your understanding of peace? What implications does this broader understanding of peace have on your daily life? Your home? Community? Your relationship with others?

Create a New Rhythm

The next time you find yourself getting anxious and your thoughts racing, stop and surrender those worries to the Lord in prayer. Take time to read Philippians 4:6-7 until you have memorized it so that you can be reminded of God's great promise of peace wherever you go.

26

Day 2 - Practicing Peace

You keep him in perfect peace whose mind is stayed on
you,
because he trusts in you.
Isaiah 26:3 (ESV)

Everyone wants peace, but few know where to find it. Some of us have looked for peace in the bottom of a bottle or the escape of a drug, to no avail. As discussed in the last lesson, true peace is only found in God. Although we may have looked elsewhere in the past to find fulfillment, those "escapes" will never satisfy or bring the healing peace we desire. God's peace fulfills us eternally, and he invites us to play an active role in experiencing his peace. God's peace is not merely a concept; it is a divine reality that we must practice in three dimensions: upward, inward, and outward.

UPWARD: Peace with God

The first step in practicing peace is to continually turn to God and receive His peace and restoration through His Son, Jesus Christ. The apostle Paul writes: "Therefore, since we have been justified by faith, we have peace with God through our Lord Jesus Christ" (Romans 5:1, ESV).

This peace, which comes from being reconciled with God the Father, is the foundation upon which all other peace is built. It is an open door, inviting us into unity and peace. The peace that comes from knowing that we are forever loved and accepted by the Creator of the universe, because of Christ's deeds. This vertical relationship sets the stage for the peace we experience inwardly and express outwardly.

INWARD: Peace Within

Jesus understands what it's like to be human. Our savior, who is very much alive and with us, experienced pain, temptation, and loss.

We read in Hebrews 4:15: "For we do not have a high priest who is unable to sympathize with our weaknesses, but one who in every respect has been tempted as we are, yet without sin" (ESV).

Because we are united with him, we share in his peace when the trials of life come our way. In Him, we live and move and have our being. If Christ is for us, and he is, who can be against us? The prophet Isaiah said, "You keep him in perfect peace whose mind is stayed on you, because he trusts in you" (Isaiah 26:3, ESV).

In the Hebrew language, the phrase "perfect peace" is "shalom shalom," literally translating to "peace of peace." This indicates an abundant, complete peace, available to those who trust in God.[13]

This isn't the absence of anxiety or fear. It is a wholeness, an anchored, deep-seated serenity that holds steady in the midst of shifting circumstances. It's not just knowing we are in Christ; it is *living in the reality* that we are inseparably united to Him, that His unchanging love is *woven into the fabric of who we are.* Though we waver and fall, our Creator remains faithful, and this truth is *etched upon our hearts.* As we entrust ourselves to Him, His peace doesn't just visit us; it *guards us*, shaping how we move through life's uncertainties with quiet surrender and holy rest.

OUTWARD: Peace Extended

Finally, the peace we receive from Christ is to be shared with others. As recipients of God's peace, we have the opportunity to be His ambassadors. We are called to be peacemakers in a world that is tearing itself apart.

This looks like sharing the good news of Jesus with those around us. This means extending grace and forgiveness instead

---

[13] Francis Brown, S.R. Driver, and Charles A. Briggs, *A Hebrew and English Lexicon of the Old Testament* (Oxford: Clarendon Press, 1907), s.v. "שׁלוֹם" (shalom).

In Hebrew, the word *shalom* (שׁלוֹם) conveys not only peace but completeness and welfare; repetition or doubling of words like *shalom shalom* can intensify the meaning, indicating "perfect peace" or "peace of peace."

of getting even. Peacemakers consider others more significant than themselves. It means being kind and compassionate, rather than harsh, and encouraging others instead of promoting ourselves. Ultimately, extending God's peace to those around us means being an imitator of Jesus.

This is your invitation to participate in God's peace. It is the gift he freely offers you. Seek peace by looking upward, by cultivating it inwardly, and by extending it outwardly. As you do, you will become a conduit of his peace to a world in desperate need of it.

* * *

Write Your Thoughts

- Nothing can separate a Christian from the love of Christ. How does this affect your sense of peace?

- We have been called to extend the peace that God has given us to others. How do you, in your personal life, extend God's peace to others?

- Write about a time when it was challenging to extend peace. Were you able to overcome the challenge and extend peace? If so, what enabled you to do it? If not, why not?

Create a New Rhythm

The next time you are wronged or mistreated by someone, remind yourself to return their malice with kindness and grace. You may be surprised how God will use this simple act of peaceful humility—for his glory, your good, and your offender's ultimate good.

27

Day 3 - Active Patience

Wait for the LORD; be strong, and let your heart take courage;
wait for the LORD!
Psalm 27:14 (ESV)

Active patience. You might be wondering, "Isn't that an oxymoron? Isn't patience, by definition, inactive? Isn't it waiting, enduring, and quietly bearing our trials?" Yet the Bible testifies otherwise. God calls us to *active engagement* rather than *passive resignation.*

Consider Joseph, a man who experienced firsthand the active nature of patience. The book of Genesis tells us how he was betrayed by his brothers, sold into slavery, wrongly accused, and then imprisoned. He had every reason to despair. But he chose to trust in the Lord, to maintain his integrity, and to serve others with diligence despite his unjust circumstances. His patience was not a weak resignation but a confident assurance

DAY 3 - ACTIVE PATIENCE

of God's faithfulness.

Joseph was in prison for two whole years for a crime he didn't commit. Most of us would have thrown up our arms in anger at God for allowing this injustice to happen to us. But Joseph possessed the foundational key to active patience: faith in God. Patience is a faith-strengthening exercise, a spiritual discipline rooted deeply in the soil of trusting in God's sovereignty and goodness.

It's crucial to understand that the substance of our faith (amount, strength, potency) is not what matters. The object of our faith is what matters: God himself. We are able to be patient because we have assurance that God is faithful, loving, and all-powerful. He is in control, and his timing is infinitely better than ours.

In the end, Joseph's faith in God was beautifully fulfilled. God had brought Joseph to prison for a perfect purpose. Joseph's faith was a light to the Egyptians, and God used Joseph to fulfill many promises to his people and display his power and love in mighty ways. We may not understand God's purposes in the moment, but we can wait patiently, daily trusting in God.

So how do we practice active patience? First and foremost, we trust God and we pray. Consider these verses: "Trust in the Lord with all your heart and do not lean on your own understanding. In all your ways acknowledge him and he will make your path straight" (Proverbs 3:5,6). "Rejoice always, pray without ceasing, give thanks in all circumstances" (1 Thessalonians 5:16-17).

The patient Christian is one who accepts the invitation to rest in God and remains in conversation with God through prayer, recognizing our dependence on Him. In prayer, we wait, knowing that while we wait, we are being refined, reshaped, and prepared for God's purposes.

As we face life's trials and tribulations, let's look to the Lord, the author and finisher of our faith. Let's choose active patience, and in doing so, resist despair, lean into hope, and witness the unfailing faithfulness of our God. Remember, his timing is perfect, his promises are sure, and his grace is sufficient.

* * *

Write Your Thoughts

- On a scale of 1-10, with 1 being "not patient at all" and 10 being "extremely patient", how would you rate your patience on average? In what areas of your life could you be more patient?

- How can we practice active patience in our day-to-day lives? If you have personal experience, please share.

- Today's reading encourages us to remember that while we wait we are being refined, reshaped, and prepared for the purposes of God. How does this perspective shift how we view periods of waiting or suffering?

Create a New Rhythm

On difficult days, make this your prayer:

Lord, grant me the grace to wait patiently, to endure faithfully, to hope expectantly. In my waiting, deepen my trust in You. Strengthen my faith and fill me with Your peace. In Jesus' name, Amen.

28

Day 4 - Patience: A "Screwtape" Letter

Be still before the Lord and wait patiently for him.
Psalm 37:7 (ESV)

Recall that *The Screwtape Letters* by C.S. Lewis is a novel in which a senior demon named "Screwtape" writes letters to his nephew, "Wormwood," a junior tempter. In his letters, Screwtape advises Wormwood on how to lead humans away from God and toward sin and death.[14]

The following letter is our version of a "Screwtape Letter." It, too, is written from the perspective of Screwtape coaching his nephew, Wormwood, in tactics to lead his human away from Christ. When the passage below refers to the "Enemy," it is referring to God. Remember, the perspective of the letter is from the demon's point of view:

---

[14] C.S. Lewis, *The Screwtape Letters* (New York: HarperCollins, 2001).

DAY 4 - PATIENCE: A "SCREWTAPE" LETTER

My Dear Wormwood,

As your older and undeniably wiser advisor, I must confess to a certain level of concern. The task before you is a formidable one, and yet, I have faith in your ability to weave the threads of discontent, anxiety, and impatience. You are to dishearten your Person from the virtue of patience—a daunting task, indeed, but a worthy one.

First, remember that in today's world, speed is everything. The humans have armed themselves with devices they call cell phones. These gadgets provide a constant stream of messages, alerts, news, and other trivial diversions—all at a moment's notice. The humans have become slaves to their devices and the bottomless hole of apps that provide them every convenience and vice.

Encourage your Person to expect this same instant gratification in all aspects of life. Foster an insatiable desire for speedy responses and immediate rewards. Let him believe that waiting is a waste of time, an outdated concept of a bygone society.

Emphasize the notion of control. Make your Person believe that through impatience—by pushing, nudging, or even bullying—he can force the world to bow to his whims. Let him feel that if he can exert enough pressure, he can master his circumstances. Remember, my dear Wormwood, that the illusion of control is one of our greatest weapons.

Convince your Person that their impatience is just a sign of productivity. If everyone else would get up to his speed, the world would be a better place. He shouldn't have to wait in lines; his time is too valuable for that. Have him fuming in anger at the gridlock traffic of his daily commute. The beauty of impatience is that it is grounded in entitlement, and entitlement is our bread and butter. Heck, my skill in entitlement tempting is what got me that bonus and the shoreline property right on the Lake of Fire!

Always remember, dear Wormwood, that the most devastating sins for your Person are the ones he doesn't know he's committing.

Your affectionate uncle,

Screwtape

***

Write Your Thoughts

- How does the concept of instant gratification, multiplied by the use of cell phones and constant access to information, contribute to the decline of patience in today's society?

- What is the relationship between our desire to be in control and our impatience?

- How can good intentions and noble goals, such as progress, hard work, and action, be twisted to justify impatience? Can you think of examples where you have justified impatience in the name of productivity?

- The phrase "time is money" is often used to justify haste and impatience. What impact does this perspective have on our lives, relationships, and spiritual well-being? Is there an alternative perspective we can adopt that values patience and deliberate action over speed?

Create a New Rhythm

Which areas of life are you the most tempted to be impatient? Take a few minutes to think about this. Pray and ask God to give you patience in those areas. In particular, ask him to teach you what it means to "Be still before the Lord and wait patiently for him" in your everyday life.

VIII

Obedience & Self-Control

*Day 1 - **Obedience: Submission to God's Authority***

*Day 2 - **Obedience From Love***

*Day 3 - **Self-Control: Sustained Obedience***

*Day 4 - **Obedience & Self-Control: A "Screwtape" Letter***

29

Day 1 - Obedience: Submission to God's Authority

If you keep my commandments, you will abide in my love, just as I have kept my Father's commandments and abide in his love. These things I have spoken to you, that my joy may be in you, and that your joy may be full.
John 15:9-11 (ESV)

We tend to think that freedom is doing whatever we want, when we want. But what if I told you true freedom is grounded in discipline? Former Navy SEAL, Jocko Willink, is famous for the counter-intuitive formula by which he lives his life: DISCIPLINE = FREEDOM. Let's explore his equation for a moment.

Willink argues that true freedom can only be experienced when we have done our duty first. Otherwise, any "freedom" we may experience is tainted by the nagging conviction that we have neglected our responsibility and we will pay for it down the road. This is why he says that discipline equals freedom. Practice his equation for a week, and I believe you'll agree that it's true. Let me take this idea one step further. I believe the truest freedom requires not only *discipline*, but *obedience* rooted in trust.

Perhaps you cringe when you hear the word "obedience." We often think of obedience as something children must practice with their parents. As adults, we balk at the idea that we need to obey anyone or anything. We don't want to feel like we are subject to anyone else's authority. Especially human authority, which can be flawed. God's authority, on the other hand, is both trustworthy and good.

In John 15:9-11, Jesus tells us that he himself obeyed his Father's commandments. He invites us to do the same, and he promises two results from this obedience. When we obey our Heavenly Father: 1) we will abide in his love and 2) our joy will be full.

God's instruction protects us from harm and creates opportunities for us to thrive. His roadmap is not designed to make life dull and bland but rather to usher in freedom from addiction and a life of true abundance. You have already practiced obedience to God to get to this point in your recovery. The key to lifelong freedom moving forward is 1) remaining obedient to God in your recovery and 2) bringing other areas of your life into obedience to God. Obedience is not merely an act of self-will, but an act of faith.

In Jesus, we have our greatest help for growing in obedience. Is there anyone who modeled this abundant life, born of obedience, more perfectly than Jesus Christ? Consider the moment in Gethsemane when Jesus, in Matthew 26:42, willingly submitted

DAY 1 - OBEDIENCE: SUBMISSION TO GOD'S AUTHORITY

to God's will, "My Father, if this cannot pass unless I drink it, your will be done." Jesus trusted his Father in obedience—even when it meant dying!

If *Discipline = Freedom*, then *Obedience = Contentment*. Obedience to God's law is not a burdensome task or an imposition on our freedoms. It's a lifeline and a guiding light that leads us to the abundant life God desires for us. The path out of addiction that leads to true life is found in following Jesus, aligning ourselves with God's will, and living within the protective walls of His commandments.

* * *

Write Your Thoughts

- In what ways have you experienced "Discipline = Freedom" or "Obedience = Contentment"?

- Obedience to God's law is about aligning with God's design for human flourishing. Can you think of an area in your life where obedience to God's commandments has led to personal growth and well-being?

- Reflecting on Jesus' prayer in Gethsemane (Matthew 26:42), how does Christ's model of obedience challenge your personal understanding and practice of submission to God's will? How can you practically apply this in your own life?

Create a New Rhythm

Choose one area of your life other than your recovery where you can begin to practice obedience to God. Ask your mentor, pastor, or friend to help you grow in this area, and to pray for your growth in this area.

30

Day 2 - Obedience from Love

There is no fear in love, but perfect love casts out fear. For fear has to do with punishment, and whoever fears has not been perfected in love. We love because he first loved us.
1 John 4:18-19 (ESV)

Imagine a beautiful day at the zoo. It's a sunny day—not too hot—and there's even a slight breeze. A father takes his two young children to see the bear exhibit. The bear, large and powerful, paces behind a glass partition. Despite the thick glass, there is a boundary line clearly marked on the floor for visitors' safety.

As they approach the exhibit, the youngest child, filled with a curious sense of bravery, inches dangerously close to the line on the floor. Observing the scene, the father gently, yet firmly, calls out to his child, "Come here, love." His voice isn't harsh or filled with anger; rather, it has a tender urgency. He's fully aware of the potential danger in his child's innocent curiosity. His call isn't meant to spoil his child's adventure but to protect her.[15]

It's the same with God. His commandments are his way of saying, "Come here, love," and flow from His profound love for us and His desire to protect us from harm. His laws aren't meant to stifle our joy or exploration of life; rather, they guide us towards safe and wholesome paths, away from the dangers we might wander into.

In the father-child relationship, *a faithful father is one who understands, one who is good, and one who has the strength to act.* The God of the Bible fits these criteria and more. Our obedience to His loving call is a reflection of our trust in His wisdom, goodness, and strength that he freely applies to us and for us; it is our recognition and response to His deep love for us.

The Apostle John reminds us of this in 1 John 4:19, "we love because He first loved us." His love is the foundation of our faith and the shining light that draws us to respond in love in return. We are only able to love him and obey him because we have experienced his amazing love for us. And the more that we experience this love through a relationship with him, the easier obedience becomes.

As we follow Jesus, obeying God out of our love for him and his love for us is a profound experience, and one we must practice and nurture. His love for us is where we find the strength and joy to obey. Abiding in his love is how we make the daily decision to choose honesty over deceit, self-control over indulgence, kindness over revenge, and generosity over greed.

Like the child who obeys a loving parent, we, too, will discover

---

[15] Adapted from a sermon illustration by Bryan Chappell.

that our obedience to our loving Heavenly Father is a path leading us to a fuller, richer life.

* * *

Write Your Thoughts

- The metaphor of the father and child at the zoo illustrates the idea that God's boundaries for us are rooted in his deep love for us. Can you think of a personal experience when you responded to God's "Come here, love" call? What was the result of obeying him?

- Have you seen your love for God lead to obedience in your life? Can you share specific examples where your love for God guided your choices?

- Which areas of your life do you need to begin obeying God the most? What has stopped you from doing so up to this point?

Create a New Rhythm

Spend a few minutes meditating on 1 John 4:19, which says, "We love because he first loved us." Ask God to help you remember this wonderful truth each day as you seek to grow in obedience to him.

31

Day 3 - Self-Control: Sustained Obedience

*A man without self-control is like a city broken into
and left without walls.*
Proverbs 25:28 (ESV)

Imagine standing in front of a massive block of ice. A sculptor approaches with tools in hand. The artist is patient and deliberate in his craft. With each disciplined strike, precise cut, and careful chip, a shape begins to emerge from the ice. Each of his movements requires the utmost concentration and control, and before long he has created a beautiful sculpture.

Before it ever rained on the earth, God gave Noah an extraordinary task. God commanded him to build an ark. This was an enormous chore, riddled with opportunities for doubts and the laughter of skeptics. But Noah did not flinch. He did not choose his way over God's. Like the careful sculptor, Noah practiced discipline and self-control—especially when his peers mocked and insulted him! His obedience to God carved out a symbol of salvation for a world on the brink of divine judgment.

Fast-forward to the garden of Gethsemane, where Jesus wrestled with the most overwhelming of circumstances. With the weight of humanity's sin on His shoulders, Jesus chose to obey the Father's will. He prayed, "My Father, if it be possible, let this cup pass from me; nevertheless, not as I will, but as you will." When he said this prayer, he mirrored the sculptor's patience, Noah's unwavering faithfulness, and their shared self-control. Despite his anguish, he chose the Father's will.

Self-control is obedience with perseverance. It is obedience in the face of temptation, fatigue, mocking, and even persecution. Jesus is the ultimate example of self-control. He was tempted in every way we are (Hebrews 4:15), yet he didn't sin. Self-control involves resisting *short-term* temptations and distractions in favor of *long-term* outcomes. As you obey God's commands and align your will with his, you will build the spiritual and moral muscle needed to resist those temptations. The more we practice obedience to God, even in the little things, the more self-control we will develop.

This relationship between obedience and self-control is beautifully reflected in Titus 2:11-12 (ESV):

> For the grace of God has appeared, bringing salvation for all people, training us to renounce ungodliness and worldly passions, and to live self-controlled, upright, and godly lives in the present age...

Paul explains here that obedience to God's grace leads us to live self-controlled lives. The Bible teaches that obedience to God is not an end in itself. It is a means through which we

DAY 3 - SELF-CONTROL: SUSTAINED OBEDIENCE

cultivate the fruit of the Spirit, one of which is self-control. This is not a burdensome command but an empowering invitation to live fully and freely. Our obedience to God's guidelines, much like the ice sculptor to the principles of his craft, shapes us to become more like Christ.

As we learn from the examples of Noah, Jesus, and the insights from Paul, obedience is more than simple compliance. It is the gateway to self-controlled, upright, and godly lives, molded and shaped by the loving hands of the Divine Potter.

***

Write Your Thoughts

- Noah's obedience required extraordinary self-control as he faced contempt, mocking, and perhaps even the temptation to doubt God. Can you recall moments in your own life when you had to exercise self-control in order to do what God was calling you to do? Or a time when your lack of self-control led to disaster? Reflect and write on one of these moments.

- In the garden of Gethsemane, Jesus chose to obey the Father's will despite His anguish. How can we draw strength from Jesus's example in our own struggles, especially when we need to exercise self-control?

- Based on Paul's teaching in Titus 2:11-12, how can the understanding of God's grace enhance our self-control? How does this play out in our daily lives as we strive to live out our faith?

- In which areas do you lack self-control? What changes can you make to begin to grow in these?

Create a New Rhythm

Choose one area of your life where you need to grow in self-control. (Ex. speech, thoughts, emotions, money, honesty, anxiety, etc.) Find a passage of Scripture that speaks to that area of weakness and memorize it.

When faced with temptation in that area, God's word will come to your aid just as Jesus resisted temptation in Matthew 4.

32

Day 4 - Obedience & Self-Control: A "Screwtape" Letter

> *By this we know that we love the children of God, when we love God and obey his commandments. For this is the love of God, that we keep his commandments.*
> *And his commandments are not burdensome.*
> 1 John 5:2-3 (ESV)

Recall that *The Screwtape Letters*, by C.S. Lewis, is a novel in which a senior demon named "Screwtape" writes letters to his nephew, "Wormwood," a junior tempter. In his letters, Screwtape advises Wormwood on how to lead humans away from God and toward sin and death.[16]

The letter below is our version of a "Screwtape Letter." It, too, is written from the perspective of Screwtape coaching his nephew, Wormwood, in tactics to lead his human away from Christ. When the passage below refers to the "Enemy," it is

---

[16] C.S. Lewis, *The Screwtape Letters* (New York: HarperCollins, 2001).

referring to God. Remember, the perspective of the letter is from the demon's point of view:

> My Dear Wormwood,
>
> I am delighted to see you embracing your role as a tempter with such enthusiasm. Yet, as your mentor, it is my duty to enhance your strategy with time-tested tactics. In our task of leading these humans astray, there is no better blueprint than Genesis 3 – the delightful disobedience of that first man and woman.
>
> Ah, such sweet rebellion, marinated in deliciously destructive pride. It leaves these humans estranged from the Enemy's plan for their lives. If only you could have been there, Wormwood! The human couple, created by the Enemy to obey His commands, rebelled when tempted with the opportunity to become like him.
>
> Now, let us address your human. You've observed his struggles with self-control, haven't you? Excellent. That is fertile ground for our work. The impulsiveness, the self-gratification, the lack of control – such human frailties are gifts to our cause! Stoke the fires of his impulsive desires, my dear nephew, and fan the flames of entitlement. Make him believe he deserves pleasure at any cost.
>
> You may also subtly suggest that he can handle more than what is set before him, especially when it comes to temptation and sin. Convince him he can

DAY 4 - OBEDIENCE & SELF-CONTROL: A "SCREWTAPE" LETTER

handle hanging out with those old friends, even if they are drinking and using.

Nurture in your human the concept of 'being the exception to the rule.' Every human wants to believe they're special, unique, above the common herd. Use this. Make him think his lack of self-control is not a flaw, but a testament to his individuality. His uniqueness makes him exempt from the Enemy's calls for obedience and self-control.

Make him believe that it is the freedom to do as he pleases that will make him happy. The more he indulges in his pride, the less he will feel the need to humble himself before the Enemy.

If your human is following the Enemy, he will develop self-control. Twist this, Wormwood. Make self-control seem a chore, a restriction on his freedom. Instead of a path to a fuller, richer life, make him see it as an obstacle to his pleasure. Make obedience a yoke, not a guide.

Your affectionate uncle,

Screwtape

* * *

Write Your Thoughts

- Given the perspective offered in the Screwtape letter and the message in 1 John 5:2-3, how are love and obedience related?

- How does this Screwtape letter depict the dangers of overestimating our abilities to resist temptation, especially when it comes to 1 Corinthians 10:13? How might we, as Christians, ensure we remain vigilant and reliant on God's strength rather than our own?

- How can the concept of being 'the exception to the rule' undermine the development of self-control and obedience? In what ways might we unintentionally fall into this trap, and how can we guard against it?

Create a New Rhythm

Cultivate a mindset of obedience to God and self-control in every area of life. Start small—how you drive to work, how you speak to coworkers, how you make space to read God's Word each day. These seemingly small acts of obedience are seeds that, when tended with care, grow into a life marked by faithfulness and lasting fruit.

IX

Love

Day 1 - **God is Love, Part 1**

Day 2 - **God is Love, Part 2: A Transformative Example**

Day 3 - **Love Your Enemies? Seriously?**

Day 4 - **Love in Action**

33

Day 1 - God is Love, Part 1

*O Lord, you have searched me and known me! You
know when I sit down and when I rise up; you discern
my thoughts from afar. You search out my path and my
lying down and are acquainted with all my ways.*
Psalm 139:1-3 (ESV)

Have you thought about the crucial role the sun plays in our lives? This massive star at the center of our solar system is the source of nearly all the energy we see and feel. Whether it is the photosynthesis in plants, the ancient energy trapped in fossil fuels, or the power in our batteries, it all ultimately stems from the sun.

The core of the sun is unimaginably hot and almost infinitely energetic. Every second, this core generates the energy equivalent of 15 billion thermonuclear fusion bombs. Yet, the sun remains intact. The tremendous gravity of the overlying gas offsets the outward push of the produced energy.[17]

The centrality of this life-giving force is not unlike God's unchanging love. Just like the sun, God's love is necessary for life to exist, and without it, nothing would flourish. And just as the sun holds our solar system together, the love of God sustains all of creation by his very word (Hebrews 1:3).

God's love is big, but it's also personal. He recognizes and understands us completely! By his words—"O Lord, you have searched me and known me!"—David reminds us of the personal nature of our relationship with God.

Theologian J.I. Packer summarized this truth when he said:

> God's love is an exercise of His goodness towards individual sinners whereby, having identified Himself with their welfare, He has given His Son to be their Savior, and now brings them to know and enjoy Him in a covenant relation.[18]

God's great love is so personal that he sent his only Son to die for the sins of his people. The beautiful union of God's perfect love and his perfect justice is displayed in full on the cross of Jesus Christ.

So what do we do with this love? Firstly, we worship in thankfulness to God. Secondly, we reflect His love to the world. Consider the moon. It doesn't produce its own light but reflects

---

[17] NASA, "Sun Facts – NASA Science," accessed June 23, 2025, https://science.nasa.gov/sun/facts/.

[18] J.I. Packer, *KnowingGod* (DownersGrove, IL: InterVarsity Press, 1973),119 (chapter 12, "The Love of God").

light from the sun. That's our role as followers of Jesus—as we experience God's love, God calls us to reflect it in our interactions with others. So, the next time you're enjoying the sunlight, think about the boundless love of God that it represents. Think of how God might use *you* to reflect that love to someone else.

* * *

Write Your Thoughts

- Can you name three ways that the sun is like God's love?

- In what ways have you personally experienced God's love in your life?

- How can you start reflecting God's love to others?

Create a New Rhythm

As noted in today's reading, the proper response to God's love on our part is to worship him. This goes beyond Sunday worship, although that's important. This means that we cultivate an attitude (or heart-posture) of adoration and thanksgiving to God for his love. Starting today, spend a few minutes every day cultivating that heart-posture of thanksgiving toward your King.

34

Day 2 - God is Love, Part 2: A Transformative Example

Anyone who does not love does not know God, because God is love.
1 John 4:8 (ESV)

Kane struggled with addiction early in his adult life. His lifestyle led him down a path of isolation and self-destruction. His addiction strained his relationships, wore down his physical health, and eroded his sense of self-worth. The world saw Kane as an addict—a failure. But then, something extraordinary happened.

God's Love: Provides Assurance
Kane became part of a recovery group that focused on God's grace and love. There, he was told about a love deeper and wider than any human love—a love that would not judge him for his addiction, failures, or shortcomings. This love came from God, and it was unwavering and unconditional. For Kane, in the

midst of his pain, this brought a sense of peace and courage he had not felt in a long time.

God's Love: Changes Self-Perception

The group helped Kane see himself not as the world saw him, but as God saw him: cherished, valuable, and capable of experiencing freedom from his addiction. This new understanding altered Kane's self-perception dramatically. He began to see a future where he was free from the clutches of addiction and could achieve great things.

God's Love: Transforms Relationships

As Kane began to understand the depth of God's love for him, his relationships began to change. He began loving others not for what they could offer him, but because he himself had experienced profound love. His relationships began to heal as he became more compassionate, understanding, and patient.

God's Love: Impacts Decision-Making

As he walked this PATH of recovery, God's love also influenced Kane's decision-making. He started making choices that reflected love, patience, authenticity, trust, and humility. His actions were not merely about staying clean but about living a life that reflected God's love to others.

God's Love: Encourages Forgiveness

Despite carrying resentment and bitterness for years, Kane found the strength to forgive — both himself and others. He began to understand that just as God forgave him despite his faults, he too could extend that same grace to others and himself. This realization was a key turning point in his recovery journey.

God's Love: Fuels Spiritual Growth

Kane's experience of God's love became the foundation of his spiritual growth. The more he jumped into God's Word, the stronger his relationship with God became. His prayer life deepened, his understanding of the Bible grew, and he developed a greater desire to serve others — especially those also struggling with addiction.

Kane's story is a composite of countless true stories we have personally observed. God's love transforms the hardest of hearts and has the power to redeem even those who feel they are too far gone.

Understanding and experiencing God's love is a lifelong journey. It can be pursued through prayer, meditation on the Scriptures, participation in a faith community, and reflecting on God's love in day-to-day life. This journey is not always easy, especially for those wrestling with addiction. However, as we continually seek God, we experience his power to transform us from the inside out. As the Apostle Paul confirms, we can be "transformed into His image with ever-increasing glory" (2 Corinthians 3:18 NIV).

God's love is the catalyst for our transformative journey from addiction to life in Christ, which is recovery in its truest sense.

* * *

Write Your Thoughts

- Where have you tried to find love or acceptance apart from

God?

- How would you describe God's love in your own words?

- Kane's story shows a complete transformation that took years to achieve. In which of the areas discussed in Kane's story do you have the farthest to go?

Create a New Rhythm

1 John 4:8 says, "Anyone who does not love does not know God, because God is love." Spend the next 3 minutes meditating on this verse. If you do not know God or believe in his great love for you, ask him to reveal Himself to you and allow you to see his goodness.

35

Day 3 - Love Your Enemies? Seriously?

You have heard that it was said, "You shall love your neighbor and hate your enemy." But I say to you, "Love your enemies and pray for those who persecute you."
Matthew 5:43-44 (ESV)

Dr. Martin Luther King Jr. was a pivotal figure in the American Civil Rights Movement. A Baptist minister by profession, Dr. King was a man of faith who sought to live by the commandment, "You shall love your neighbor as yourself." He devoted his life to serving his community, striving for equality and justice.

Jesus taught in the Sermon on the Mount to "love your enemies and pray for those who persecute you." The American Civil Rights Movement provided many opportunities to practice Jesus' teachings. One poignant example is Dr. King's response to the violence his followers faced during the Montgomery Bus

Boycott in 1956. When his home was bombed in retaliation for his leadership in the boycott, Dr. King remained calm and insisted on a nonviolent response. He addressed an angry crowd outside his home, urging them to "go home and say a prayer for the people who committed this act." Even in the face of direct and personal attacks, Dr. King chose to meet his enemies with love.

Perhaps most notably, in his "Loving Your Enemies" sermon delivered at Dexter Avenue Baptist Church in Montgomery, Alabama, King directly addressed this Biblical teaching. He urged his listeners to discover the "redemptive power of love," saying, "When you rise to the level of love, of its great beauty and power, you seek only to defeat evil systems. Individuals who happen to be caught up in that system, you love, but you seek to defeat the system."

How was Dr. King even able to get to a place where he could attempt to love his enemy? *Because his love was not powered by feelings he had to stir up from within himself.* Dr. King had just as many flaws as most of us, but he did not forget that "We love because he first loved us" - 1 John 4:19 (*ESV*). God is the one who empowers us to love our enemies.

* * *

Write Your Thoughts

- Reflecting on the commandments in Matthew 5:43-44 and Matthew 22:37, how might you practice this in your life?

- Have you ever been loved by an enemy? Have you ever loved your enemy? Describe what happened in these events.

- Name someone that you find hard to love or forgive in your life. What is holding you back from loving them?

Create a New Rhythm

The next time you are faced with someone you would consider an enemy or someone you resent, offer them love instead of hatred. We must make a habit of loving our enemies if we are to follow Jesus. After all, while we were God's enemies, he sent his Son to die for us.

36

Day 4 - Love in Action

Two others, who were criminals, were led away to be put to death with him. And when they came to the place that is called The Skull, there they crucified him, and the criminals, one on his right and one on his left. And Jesus said, "Father, forgive them, for they know not what they do." And they cast lots to divide his garments. And the people stood by, watching, but the rulers scoffed at him, saying, "He saved others; let him save himself, if he is the Christ of God, his Chosen One!"
Luke 23:33-35 (ESV)

This vivid scene from the Gospel of Luke is chilling when you think about it. The Son of God, who has done nothing wrong, is murdered like a common criminal in front of jeering crowds that mock him as he suffers. Added to the physical pain of his crucifixion is the embarrassment of being stripped, tortured, and executed in front of the populace of the largest city in his country, all while his friends and family look on helplessly.

Jesus' crucifixion is the greatest injustice that has ever happened or will ever happen. He lived a sinless life, yet he was condemned. He committed no crime, yet he was punished. He did nothing to cause him shame—and to me, this is one of the most haunting realities of the cross—yet he willingly took on the unbearable weight of all of our shame.

The Bible says that "For our sake he made him to be sin who knew no sin, so that in him we might become the righteousness of God" (2 Corinthians 5:21 ESV). The idea that God himself would take on the guilt of sin to save his creation is so unjust that it should never have happened! And yet, praise be to God for his steadfast love!

Just before he was taken to be killed, Jesus told his disciples, "Greater love has no one than this, that someone lay down his life for his friends" (John 15:13 ESV). Jesus' life wasn't taken, it was *given*—and it was given *for you*. There is no greater example of love than Jesus. His entire earthly life was the living embodiment of perfect love for God and others. This is seen nowhere more clearly than at the climax of all of history, his crucifixion. Jesus himself is love in action.

So what now? The very next words out of Jesus' mouth were, "You are my friends if you do what I command you" (John 15:14 ESV). Because he loves us, we take action!

* * *

Write Your Thoughts

- What stands out to you about Luke 23:33-35?

- According to 2 Corinthians 5:21 listed above, what is the reason that Jesus died?

- In light of what Jesus has done for you, what action do you think God is calling you to take?

Create a New Rhythm

Take 15 minutes to get away from distractions and be by yourself. Read Luke 23:26-43, but not quickly like you might your favorite novel. Instead, read it slowly and with emotion as you would read the obituary of a family member. Meditate on the events described in the text. Let your heart respond to God from what you read.

X

Worship & Christian Community

*Day 1 - **Worship: The Rhythm of Recovery***

*Day 2 - **The Lord's Day***

*Day 3 - **All of Life as Worship***

*Day 4 - **Together***

37

Day 1 - Worship: The Rhythm of Recovery

Let us hold fast the confession of our hope without wavering, for he who promised is faithful. And let us consider how to stir up one another to love and good works, not neglecting to meet together, as is the habit of some, but encouraging one another, and all the more as you see the Day drawing near.
Hebrews 10:23-25 (ESV)

There is considerable confusion about worship these days. Is worship singing church music? Is worship enjoying God in our hearts? Is it bowing before God and honoring him? Is it supposed to be boring? Is it supposed to be fun? Is it about God? Is it about me? Is it one day a week? Or is it every day? You can answer "yes" to almost all of these questions. But I prefer this definition: *true worship is God's designed pathway for us to draw near to him in adoration.*

It is no exaggeration to say that worship is the central and essential piece that brings all of the chapters of this book together. All of the things we've been talking about—Honesty, Humility, Repentance, Gratitude, Forgiveness, Spiritual Disciplines, Peace, Patience, Self-Control, Obedience, and Love—are elements found in worship. They are enacted, experienced, practiced, trained, encouraged, and shared in worship.

This workbook is called *Rhythms of Recovery*, and worship is THE rhythm of recovery. It is the heartbeat of a new life that has been transformed. Because of this, we MUST gather together with the people of God and worship the Lord according to his design on the Lord's Day.

From the moment of Creation, in the very structure of the Garden in Eden and the placement of the Tree of Life, God designed the rhythms of relationship with Him to meet the needs of his image-bearing creatures. We are made to draw near and worship God, to know him, to be known by him, and enjoy him. Part of knowing him is giving ourselves to him and receiving his gifts.

Because worship isn't just about giving, but also receiving.

I confess that, for much of my life, I saw worship as a chore. Going to church on Sunday to worship seemed boring or irrelevant. The truth is, I didn't understand what worship was or why we worship God. I missed the beauty of the relationship God was graciously offering to me, and in my selfishness, I only wanted what *I* thought would "benefit" me. I didn't realize that worship *does* benefit me. As we give and, in turn, receive from God in worship, we are transformed.

How are we transformed? The rhythm of regular worship transforms us. By humbling ourselves before God, we allow the Holy Spirit to transform our hearts. As our hearts are transformed, we increasingly abide in Christ, and he uses us to shine a powerful light on those around us. We give praise to God because he is worthy of all praise and glory, and in return, we receive gifts from him as we draw near to his throne in worship. What kind of gifts? Here's a short list:

- Becoming more like Christ in character (love, joy, peace, patience, kindness, goodness, faithfulness, gentleness, and self-control)[19]
- Growing in love and affection for God
- And receiving true peace that only God can give (Phil 4:6-7)

When we surrender ourselves to God in worship, we open our hearts to receive all these things and more.

The bottom line is that we are made to meet with God in worship. When we see how God calls us to Himself and meets the needs of our hearts, we can't help but become hungry for more. We begin to gladly confess our sins and unload our burdens as we hear and receive the gospel proclamation of grace and forgiveness. We begin to be glad for the instruction and encouragement from God through the preaching of his Word, to feast with him at his table, and to receive the good word of benediction (blessing).

In other words, worship is a response. Not just an outward response, but an inward heart response. It's our heart's response to his unwavering love, his rich mercy, his abundant grace, and more. When our heart is worshiping, it overflows into every aspect of our lives.

We did not initiate this relationship; God did out of his great

---

[19] Galatians 5:22-23 (English Standard Version).

love for us. "We love because he first loved us" (1 John 4:19 ESV). This statement alone should draw us to Him, in love. As we continually give him the praise, glory, devotion, and honor he deserves, our experience of his love and grace is taken to new heights, and his transforming power is displayed in our lives.

* * *

Write Your Thoughts

- What does it mean to you to draw near to God? Is that something you are excited about or apprehensive about?

- What assumptions and expectations do you bring to worship?

- Have you ever been blessed by worshiping the Lord? If so, please explain.

DAY 1 - WORSHIP: THE RHYTHM OF RECOVERY

Create a New Rhythm

Think about one way that you can incorporate worship in your recovery—in attitude, or action. Share your goal with your mentor/group and ask for accountability to follow through. Examples:

1. Get plugged in at a local church
2. Volunteer to serve others
3. Intentionally practice gratitude to God on the way to work

Write your goal here:

38

Day 2 - The Lord's Day

Let the word of Christ dwell in you richly, teaching and admonishing one another in all wisdom, singing psalms and hymns and spiritual songs, with thankfulness in your hearts to God.
Colossians 3:16 (ESV)

You may be asking yourself, "What exactly is 'the Lord's Day'?" The Lord's Day refers to a day of the week—typically Sunday—that we regularly set aside for the worship of God. The title "The Lord's Day" comes from Revelation 1:10, where the apostle John says, "I was in the Spirit on the Lord's day, and I heard behind me a loud voice like a trumpet" (ESV).

The Lord's Day has six primary elements, as described in various passages throughout the Bible:

- Singing Psalms, hymns, and spiritual songs
- The preaching of God's Word

- Prayer
- Giving of tithes and offerings
- The sacraments
- Fellowship

Let's take a look at each one.

Singing (Hebrews 12:28)

This is what most of us tend to think of as worship. The songs that we sing should exalt God for who he is and what he has done. They should be primarily about him, not us. They should draw inspiration from Scripture. For thousands of years, Christians have sung the Psalms, and so can you!

Preaching

The preaching of God's Word is how he speaks to his people. It is crucial that the preaching is from the Bible, is Christ-centered, and lines up with the rest of Scripture. The result of good preaching is 1) God is glorified, 2) you are convicted of sin, 3) you are encouraged by your Savior, 4) you have a deeper understanding of the biblical text, and 5) you are equipped and empowered to take the Gospel to the world. The next time you are sitting there listening to a sermon, picture the Lord standing behind your pastor and speaking through him.

Prayer

Like singing, prayer is an act of going before God's throne. When we pray as a congregation, we are praising him, thanking him, and petitioning him as a family of believers. When we pray, our attitude should be solemn, our mind should be focused, and our heart should be bowed in reverence to the King.

Giving (Proverbs 3:9, 2 Corinthians 9:7, Deuteronomy 14:22-29)

All of our possessions, including our money, belong to God. As his stewards, he asks that we manage them wisely. The word "tithe" means "tenth," and in the Old Testament, people gave one-tenth of what they made to God every year. There is a very strong argument that we should keep practicing the tithe today.

When you give to your local church or other worthy ministry, be generous! Give "off the top," before you give to Caesar—another way of saying before taxes, not after. Do you want a net blessing or a gross blessing? Giving with a cheerful heart is an act of worship in itself.

Sacraments

There are two sacraments: baptism and the Lord's Supper. Both of these were instituted by Jesus himself to be practiced by his people when they gather together. Baptism is the sign of the new covenant, just as circumcision was the sign of the old covenant. It is an outward sign of the inward reality that you have been born again and your sins have been forgiven because Jesus paid for them on the cross.

Jesus instituted the Lord's Supper on the night he was betrayed. As he sat with his disciples, he gave them bread and wine, saying, "This is my body," and "This is my blood of the covenant, which is poured out for the forgiveness of sins" (Matthew 26:26-28 ESV). When we partake of the Lord's Supper today, we are doing so in remembrance of Jesus and his sacrifice for us. The apostle Paul tells us that "as often as you eat this bread and drink the cup, you proclaim the Lord's death until he comes" (1 Corinthians 11:26 ESV).

Fellowship

DAY 2 - THE LORD'S DAY

Have you ever been outside in a snowstorm? The biting cold, blinding snow, and relentless wind can be overwhelming. But when you finally make it indoors, the warmth and light melt away your despair.

Going to church should feel like that. By simply spending time together as a group of believers, we encourage one another in our faith. If church doesn't feel like that for you, here is a secret: it didn't for anyone else the first time they went to church. *The secret to developing deep fellowship and friendship at church is simple: keep showing up!*

For so many of us, Sunday is the day that we become depressed that the weekend is over and another week of work and toil is about to begin. But Sunday ought to be the Everest of our week, with the worship service being the summit. Everything builds to that moment when we are praising God together, energized to go and serve God for another week.

* * *

Write Your Thoughts

- Which part of the Lord's Day is your favorite, and why?

- Which part of the Lord's Day do you find the most challenging, and why?

- Do you consistently go to church each week? If not, why not?

- What change can you make to deepen your worship on the Lord's Day?

Create a New Rhythm

Make it a habit to attend Sunday worship service faithfully. This is where you have the opportunity to go before the throne of the God of the universe in praise. This is where you are fed from the preaching of God's Word. This is where you can fellowship with brothers and sisters in Christ who can encourage you in your walk with Jesus, and you can do the same for them!

Do this for one year, and you will never be the same person again. Put this to the test and watch God transform your heart.

39

Day 3 - All of Life as Worship

I appeal to you therefore, brothers, by the mercies of God, to present your bodies as a living sacrifice, holy and acceptable to God,
which is your spiritual worship.
Romans 12:1-2 (ESV)

The apostle Paul tells us that we ought to present our bodies as a living sacrifice to God. In the context of scripture, a sacrifice was typically an animal that had been killed, so it would be unusual for Paul to speak of a living sacrifice. What does he mean?

If we look at Paul's life, one thing is clear: *Paul practiced what he preached.* He didn't speak empty words, but he lived out radical obedience. He was relentless in his pursuit of Christ's call on his life, and his intense dedication came at a great cost. While on his missionary journeys, Paul was shipwrecked, beaten, and imprisoned multiple times because of his faith in

Christ.

On one occasion, in Acts 14, Paul entered the town of Lystra (now in present-day Turkey) and boldly preached the Gospel there. God was using him in powerful ways, and it was creating quite a commotion! The Jews from a neighboring city caught wind that Paul and Barnabas were in Lystra teaching about Jesus, and they devised a plan to have Paul killed.

The Jews went to Lystra, bringing with them angry crowds that they had stirred up against Paul. In no time, the local Lystrians were swept into the angry mob, and they violently stoned Paul, pelting him with heavy rocks until they thought he was dead. Then they dumped his body outside the city.

When Paul came to, he brushed himself off and *went back into the city!* Gathering his followers, he went to the nearby city of Derbe and preached the Gospel there. After making many disciples there, Paul, Barnabas, and their followers returned, not just to Lystra where Paul was almost killed, but also to Antioch and Iconium, the cities from which the angry crowds of Jews had originally come!

Paul preached the Gospel again in all three cities as if the people hadn't tried to kill him there. Many were healed and came to trust Christ, resulting in the establishment of multiple churches in these cities. They went from killing Paul (or so they thought) to calling him brother. Paul rightly viewed his life as forfeit for the sake of his King. In his own words:

> I have been crucified with Christ. It is no longer I who live, but Christ who lives in me. And the life I now live in the flesh I live by faith in the Son of God, who loved me and gave himself for me.

DAY 3 - ALL OF LIFE AS WORSHIP

> Galatians 2:20 (ESV)

And again,

> For to me to live is Christ, and to die is gain.
> Philippians 1:21 (ESV)

God might ask you to do some hard things, things that might not be safe. Trusting him is an act of worship. Worship is not just a Sunday service; it is a way of life. Our truest, deepest worship is surrendering the thing we hold most dear: our very life.

We worship God in the way we pursue a relationship with him, the intentionality we put into our recovery, and the diligence we practice in our daily work. God receives the glory when we are obedient to him, and that is true whether we are being persecuted like Paul or simply choosing to show kindness rather than bitterness or selfishness.

Why should we worship God in every aspect of our lives? The reality is that we are always worshiping or "serving" something or someone. Most of the time, our object of worship is ourselves. But whether we are worshiping ourselves, others, things, or ideas, *the only master who can fulfill our desires is the living God who created us.* He is the only one who can love us perfectly and fill that empty pit of longing in our hearts.

There are countless reasons why we should worship God, but the core reason is this: As the Creator of the universe who designed and formed all things and who is ever-present with abounding grace and love for his children, only God is worthy of our constant and life-long worship; only God can fulfill our deepest desires and needs and give us abundant life, peace, hope, and joy.

What a promise! Truly, no person, idea, promise, dream, substance, or thing can be a better master than the living God of the Bible.

> *So, whether you eat or drink, or whatever you do,*
> *do all to the glory of God.*
> 1 Corinthians 10:31 (ESV)

* * *

Write Your Thoughts

- What do you think it means to "present your bodies as a living sacrifice, holy and acceptable to God"?

- Would you say that worship is a regular rhythm of life for you? Why or why not?

- What are some ways that you can worship God in your daily

life?

Create a New Rhythm

Today in America, we rarely face extreme persecution for Jesus like our martyr brothers and sisters of the past. However, we each have the opportunity every day to eat, drink, live, and work for God's glory. This Rhythm is the ultimate Rhythm: *to become a living sacrifice of worship to your King in all that you do.*

Not sure where to start? Scripture tells us how to do this. Read God's word, and ask him to reveal Himself to you. Examine your heart and your actions. Today and every day, cultivate this rhythm of seeking to live your life in a way that honors and glorifies the Most High God in all that you do.

40

Day 4 - Together

And though a man might prevail against one who is alone, two will withstand him— a threefold cord is not quickly broken.
Ecclesiastes 4:12 (ESV)

Every year that I played sports in high school, our coaches would come up with a motto for the season. This motto served as a theme to focus on throughout the season, uniting and bonding us as a team. They would print the motto on our practice shirts, on the wall in the weight room, and throughout the locker room.

My freshman year, the theme was one word: "together." This theme word, along with a Bible verse, was printed on our warm-up jersey. The verse they chose was Ecclesiastes 4:12 (which you'll find at the top of this page). Our coaches taught us that we could only win games against determined opponents if we did it as one unit, together.

DAY 4 - TOGETHER

The same is true of recovery and the Christian life. *We can only succeed together.* In Acts 2:42-47, we find a detailed description of what life looked like in the early church. It is called "the early church" because the events of Acts 2 took place right on the heels of Jesus' death, resurrection, and ascension.

Here is what life looked like for members of the early church:

- They devoted themselves to God's Word
- They embraced fellowship with each other
- They shared resources with those in need
- They praised God with gratitude
- God saved more souls every day
- All those who believed were together

There is a saying I used to hear a lot in the recovery meetings I went to: "*I* drink, *we* recover." This saying illustrates how we become bound by the chains of addiction through isolation and selfishness. Conversely, we experience freedom and long-term recovery by cultivating a healthy community through vulnerability and selflessness toward others.

Consider the following formulas:

1. Isolation + Temptation + Time = Relapse

This formula is solid. I can't tell you how many times I have seen this play out both in my own life and in the lives of those we serve at Unbound Grace.

2. Healthy Community + Temptation + Time = Resilience

The key to this formula is a proper understanding of having a "healthy community."

As we mentioned, to be in a healthy community, you must be vulnerable. That means you can be honest with at least one other person in your community about your past and your current struggles. The "resilience" in this formula stems from facing temptation without giving in to it. There is no better model for us in this than Jesus in Matthew 4.

Worship is the heartbeat of biblical community. As you strive to worship God in every aspect of your life, you will be amazed at how the Lord rewards your obedience by meeting all of your needs—especially by supplying brothers and sisters to walk alongside you.

* * *

Write Your Thoughts

- Share a time in your life when doing something "together" with someone else was better than doing it alone.

- List three characteristics of the early church in Acts 2. Which of these seems the hardest for us to do today?

- How would you describe your community right now? Is it healthy? Are you isolated? Are there people bringing you down instead of building you up?

- What can you do to improve your community right now?

Create a New Rhythm

Think of one way that you can improve your community right now and put it into action. Some examples may include:

- Commit to join a new small group, recovery group, or church meeting.
- Reach out to a family member or friend and invite them to get together every week (rain or shine) as part of your weekly routine.
- Find an opportunity to serve someone less fortunate than you who might need someone to talk to on a regular basis. (Nursing homes are great for this!)

Joining a new group can feel awkward at first, but don't let that discourage you! Be consistent and show up. You will be amazed at what God will do in your life.

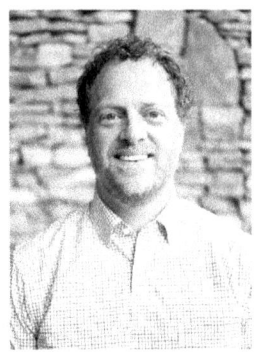

About the Author

JOHN STEAKLEY, M.Div., BCPC, is certified in addiction and mental health recovery and the founder of Unbound Grace Ministries—a Christ-centered counseling ministry dedicated to guiding individuals and families through the challenges of addiction and other struggles. With a focus on spiritual health, relational connection, and lasting transformation, Unbound Grace offers compassionate, clinically informed care rooted in the hope of the Gospel.

John was born in Dallas, Texas, grew up in Huntsville, Alabama, and has lived in Birmingham, Alabama, since 2005. A graduate of the University of Alabama and Beeson Divinity School, he turned the challenges of his own addiction into a lifeline for others by founding Unbound Grace Ministries in 2018. For over a decade, John served on staff as a pastor in Birmingham, but it's in his current role as a pastoral counselor that he's found his calling: guiding souls through the wilderness of addiction and toward hope and healing. His unique blend of spiritual guidance, evidence-based therapy, and real-world application has touched countless lives.

Married with two lively daughters (and a dog named Bear), John is a living testament that transformation is attainable through God's grace. The core of his work lies in the belief that recovery is not just possible, it's a divine gift. Visit the Unbound Grace website to learn more about the unique approach of this ministry or to inquire about John's availability for speaking and preaching engagements.

You can connect with me on:
🌐 https://unboundgrace.life

Also by John Steakley

John has also written a book about his own journey to find hope and freedom from the chains of addiction. You can purchase copies of his book on Amazon.com.

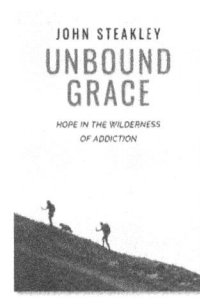

Unbound Grace: Hope in the Wilderness of Addiction

It is desire's nature to want more. No human is free from this predicament, and, as a result, we are all addicts in need of recovery. After rehab, when John Steakley's battle with substance and alcohol addiction really began, he discovered that true recovery was impossible without help. This deep truth applies to everyone.

Unbound Grace addresses the deeper issues of addiction by

- Exploring how to understand better who you are and where you find belonging

- Examining God's story and who he is

- Reconciling how your story fits into God's restoration story for humanity

Each chapter presents an illustration and explores the problem, suggests a plan to address it, illuminates the path to restoration, and offers useful tools to collect as your recovery progresses. This book is not just for those struggling with addictions; it's for anyone who admits they need help understanding how Christ loves them and what that means in their everyday life.

www.ingramcontent.com/pod-product-compliance
Lightning Source LLC
Chambersburg PA
CBHW060317050426
42449CB00011B/2528